HEALTHY SKIN

HEALTHY SKIN

A GUIDE TO LIFELONG SKIN CARE

RICHARD A. WALZER, M.D.,

AND THE EDITORS OF CONSUMER REPORTS BOOKS

Consumers Union

Mount Vernon, New York

ISBN 0-89043-266-X

Designed by Susan Hood
Drawings by John W. Karapelou
First printing, September 1989
Manufactured in the United States of America

Photo credits for color insert appearing between pages 148 and 149 are as follows: Lyme disease—courtesy of Pfizer Central Research (left) and U.S. Centers for Disease Control (right). Malignant melanoma—photos reproduced with permission of The Skin Cancer Foundation, New York, N.Y., from the brochure "The Many Faces of Malignant Melanoma," copyright © 1985, 1987.

Originally published in 1981 by Appleton-Century-Crofts under the title *Skintelligence*. This edition has been revised and updated.

To my wife, Joyce

CONTENTS

INTRODUCTION   1

1: ABOUT THE SKIN   5
2: DERMATITIS   13
3: PSORIASIS   31
4: ACNE   36
5: SKIN ALLERGIES   51
6: THE SKIN AND NUTRITION   71
7: THE HAIR AND NAILS   81
8: THE LIPS AND MOUTH   105
9: SKIN INFECTIONS AND SEXUALLY TRANSMITTED
    DISEASES   113
10: BITES AND STINGS   134
11: THE SUN AND SKIN CANCER   143
12: MOLES AND OTHER BENIGN SKIN GROWTHS   156
13: SKIN PIGMENTATION   164
14: PEDIATRIC SKIN PROBLEMS   175
15: THE PSYCHE AND THE SKIN   190
16: DERMATOLOGICAL COSMETIC PROCEDURES   198

A BRIEF GLOSSARY   205
APPENDIX: SKIN PRODUCT RATINGS   209
INDEX   233

HEALTHY SKIN

INTRODUCTION

For years dermatologists have been accused of practicing the art of medicine while ignoring its science. But in the past three decades, when most branches of medical science made significant gains, the field of dermatology did not lag behind. Quite the contrary. There has been an explosion of study and research, the results of which are now evident. Recent developments in skin medications and allied technology have permanently altered the treatment and prognosis of many chronic skin problems. Today's dermatologists can claim a comprehensive, if not complete, understanding of the behavior of normal skin and the cause of most skin disorders.

Unfortunately, many old concepts still prevail and are reflected in the articles and books written for the education of the public. This book attempts to present a concise, objective overview of the field of contemporary dermatology. As much as possible, the established facts are allowed to speak for themselves, and subjects that defy understanding are not further obscured with convenient but possibly false explanations. This book is not meant to be all-inclusive, but it does provide information about most common skin problems.

Selecting a Dermatologist

There are many well-trained dermatologists in the United States who are certified by the American Board of Dermatology.

1

Many of these physicians have training and expertise in other medical specialties such as internal medicine, pediatrics, allergy, and surgery. With the expansion of residency training programs in recent years, dermatologists can be found in many more smaller communities and on the staffs of local hospitals.

If dermatologists are readily available and their competence can be confirmed by the referring physician, a local medical society, medical directories, or reliable friends and former patients, then what other factors should you consider? The doctor's personality, medical philosophy, and expertise in an area relevant to your particular needs are three important areas.

Fortunately, most patients are able to accommodate themselves to a range of medical personalities and styles as long as there is compatibility with the physician's medical philosophy and his or her convictions about such matters as the use of medications and other forms of therapy, and the importance of laboratory tests and specialty consultations. A medical philosophy also takes in office management style: personnel, appointment schedules, fees and insurance claims, to mention but a few areas of potential doctor-patient conflict.

Another area of difference may be the extent of the doctor's willingness to communicate with the patient about all aspects of diagnosis and treatment. This factor is especially important in the field of dermatology, where the dermatologist must set realistic goals for the patient in regard to various types of therapy. Frankness and candor on the part of the doctor are essential, for instance, when treating chronic skin disorders such as psoriasis, atopic dermatitis (eczema), and acne. If the doctor does not provide the patient with realistic expectations, the patient is likely to be sorely disappointed with the care he or she receives.

Some prospective patients are looking for a "super-specialist," a dermatologist who specializes in a particular area of dermatology. For such patients there are pediatric dermatologists, allergy-oriented dermatologists, dermatopathologists, and dermatological surgeons, to say nothing of dermatologists with a special interest in diseases such as psoriasis, atopic dermatitis, blistering diseases, and skin cancer. How do you find a super-specialist? If your local medical society or community dermatologist cannot provide you with referral information, write or call the American Academy of Dermatology, 1567 Maple Avenue, P.O. Box 3116, Evanston, Illinois 60204-3116, telephone (312) 869-3954.

Of all the subspecialists in dermatology, it is the dermatological surgeons, particularly the cosmetic surgeons, who are most sought after by patients. The criteria for selecting a dermatological surgeon would include technical competence and honesty at the top of the list. Most cosmetic surgeons, for instance, are happy to provide prospective patients with complete information about probable results and the potential pitfalls of a procedure. If the patient is dissatisfied with the results, both patient and doctor are losers. Unfortunately, the popular media tend to glorify cosmetic surgical procedures, concentrating too much on dazzling results and downplaying the frequently mediocre-to-poor consequences, as well as any potential for undesirable side effects. This often leads people to have distorted and unrealistic expectations about cosmetic surgery.

Again, for any skin problem or procedure, select a dermatologist or a dermatological specialist who has good medical qualifications, is recommended to you as competent and knowledgeable, and who agrees with you about significant areas of medical philosophy. In general, it's best to ask your general practitioner or internist, or other doctors with whom you have a satisfying medical relationship, for these recommendations.

The Ratings Charts

Consult the appendix of this book for *Consumer Reports* Ratings on a variety of skin and hair products. Ratings of individual brands are based on CU's laboratory tests, controlled-use tests, surveys, and/or expert judgments. Although the Ratings are not an infallible guide, they do offer comparative buying information that can greatly increase the likelihood that you will receive value for your money.

The information contained herein concerning brand names and formulations was originally published in *Consumer Reports* magazine—the date of the original article is noted on each Ratings chart. Please keep in mind that product names and formulas may change from time to time.

3

1 ABOUT THE SKIN

The questions that are asked of dermatologists often reflect a lack of understanding about the normal functions of this organ. Questions such as, "Do we shed our skin every two years?" or, "Are there seven layers to the skin?" cry out for more than a simple yes or no answer. The discussion that follows will provide some basic facts about the anatomy and function of the skin that should help answer these and other common queries. This information will be helpful, although not essential, for an understanding of the chapters that follow.

The skin is the largest organ system of the body, both in surface area and in weight. In the average-sized man, the skin covers some two square yards and weighs more than ten pounds. The thickness of the skin varies from approximately one-half of a millimeter in thin areas such as the eyelid, to more than two millimeters on the very thick-skinned palms and soles. (There are approximately twenty-five millimeters in one inch.)

THE STRUCTURE OF THE SKIN

From an anatomical point of view, skin can be considered to be a two-layered structure. There are, however, subdivisions within these layers. The outermost tissue is called the *epidermis*

5

and beneath it is the *dermis*. The layer of fat under the dermis is referred to as the *subcutaneous tissue* (see Figure 1).

Although the epidermis is only paper-thin, it is composed of more than twenty layers of cells, including dead cells. The function of these cells has been aptly described by the phrase "born to die." New epidermal cells that are created through cells dividing in the lowest, or basal, cell layer ascend to the skin surface, where they assume a short-lived protective function and are then imperceptibly shed from the body. During this passage, which takes approximately four weeks, the epidermal cells undergo a unique change in their composition and structure, a process called *keratinization*. From living, metabolically functioning cells, they gradually change into flat, lifeless cells composed of the complex protein substance called *keratin* (see Figure 2).

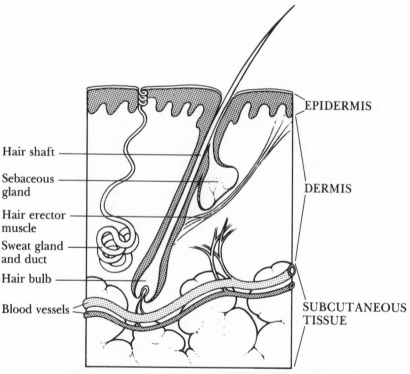

Figure 1. Cross section of the skin

It is the unique properties of keratin that provide many of the protective functions of the skin. Keratin not only serves as a barrier to physical and chemical injury, but it also provides a protective covering membrane that helps to maintain the body's internal balance by preventing water and other essential materials from escaping into the external environment.

The still-living cells found between the basal cells and the outer keratin layer are called *spiny cells*, because they appear to be bound to each other by spinelike bridges. Although these cells are tightly knit together in healthy skin, there are many diseases that can interrupt this network.

The *melanocyte* is another important cell found interspersed throughout the basal cell layer of the epidermis. This cell synthesizes *melanin*, a darkly pigmented material that lends color to the skin. The normal and abnormal functions of the melanocyte are discussed in detail in a later section on disorders of pigmentation (see chapter 13).

The epidermis is attached to the underlying layer of the der-

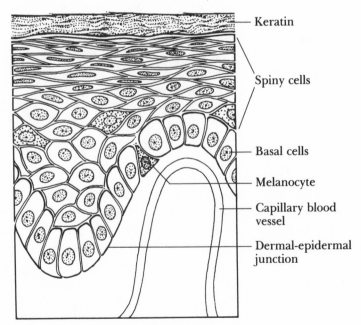

Figure 2. The cells of the epidermis

mis by complex structures and forces. This area is called the *dermal-epidermal junction* (see Figure 2). It is a critical site where nutrients and oxygen leave the small capillary blood vessels of the dermis to supply nourishment to the epidermal cells. When a disease or injury affects this sensitive junction area, the epidermis separates from the dermis and a blister appears on the skin surface. A few hard sets of tennis can provide sufficient trauma to the foot or hand to cause a dermal-epidermal separation, as can some serious skin diseases.

The dermis itself is made up of connective tissue that is a mixture of water, gel-like materials, and elastic and collagen fibers. The semi-solid nature of the dermis provides the skin with strength, suppleness, and elasticity, and it is these properties that are lost as the skin ages. The aging process is characterized by a gradual reduction in the number and thickness of the connective tissue fibers. This is perceived from the outside as a loss of texture, firmness, and elastic rebound. These combined changes are responsible for the wrinkling phenomenon. How much of the wrinkling is due to ultraviolet light and how much to aging is a matter of conjecture. However, sun damage is essential for most so-called aging to occur.

In addition to the connective tissue elements, the dermis contains blood vessels, lymph channels, nerve fibers, and even muscle cells. But it is the hair follicles, the sebaceous glands, and the sweat glands that make the skin a distinctive organ.

THE HAIR

The *hair follicle* is similar to the epidermis in that its major function is to manufacture a keratin structure, in this case, the hair itself. Hair follicles are distributed over the entire body with the exception of the palms and soles. Not all follicles, however, are actively making hairs. In many areas, the hairs that are produced are rather fine compared to the thick, heavily pigmented hairs found on the scalp and in the male beard. The fine, lighter hairs that grow on the body are called *vellus hairs*. They also appear as the end-stage hairs on the otherwise shiny domes of men with male-pattern baldness (see chapter 7).

The structure of the hair follicle is complicated. A simplified version is described and illustrated in the diagram (Figure 3). The deepest portion of the hair follicle is called the hair bulb, and it is composed of a cluster of dividing epidermal cells that surround a ball of connective tissue, blood vessels, and nerve fibers called the *papillae*. The hair papilla is the root or, rather, the nerve center of the follicle. This structure is singularly sensitive to the various injuries and diseases that can affect the growth of the hair. (Falling scalp hair found on the comb or in the skin may have an expanded, bulbous portion at the end of the hair shaft. This is not the papilla or hair root, but merely an enlarged portion of the already dead hair shaft.)

In a manner that is quite similar to the keratinization of the skin, cells in the hair bulb divide and ascend to the skin surface, turning into keratin in the process. The portion of the hair shaft that can be seen projecting from the opening of the hair follicles is completely keratinized and therefore lifeless. A spe-

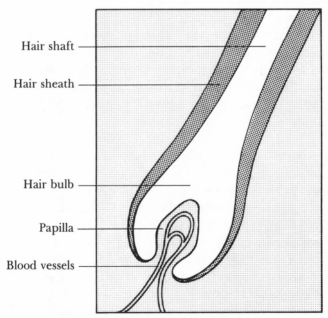

Figure 3. Cross section of a hair

cial type of muscle fiber attached to the hair follicle can quite literally make the hair stand on end, a condition known as "goose bumps."

The *sebaceous glands* (shown in Figure 1) are attached to the hair follicles by a hollow tube of cells. These glands manufacture sebum, an oily substance that reaches the skin surface via the hair follicle, where it provides a lubricating and protective film. Sebaceous glands are found throughout the skin except for the palms and soles. In several areas of the body the hair follicles are tiny, but the sebaceous glands attached to them are large and overly generous producers of skin oil. The face, back, and chest, the primary sites of acne, are areas where the size of the sebaceous glands overshadows the rather small hair follicles.

THE SWEAT GLANDS

There are two distinctive sweat-secreting skin structures: the *eccrine* and the *apocrine* glands. The apocrine glands are found under the arms, in the skin around the nipples, and in the genital and perianal areas. These primitive sweat glands are a throwback to our four-legged progenitors. In animals, apocrine glands produce a secretion, the odor of which sends out a message of identification to friends and enemies and which, at appropriate times, also attracts potential mates. In human beings, apocrine glands appear to serve no useful function. In fact, they are best known for their unpleasant qualities, since apocrine sweat is responsible for body odor. Although apocrine sweat is a sterile and odorless solution when it arrives on the skin surface, the presence of bacteria living on the axillary or underarm area of the skin changes the chemical nature of the sweat and produces a pungent odor.

The term *bromhidrosis* is used to describe a condition where there is a marked exaggeration of normal body odor. The unpleasant smell can be so overwhelming that it lingers in a room long after the person with this condition has left. Although there is no cure for bromhidrosis, the most effective measure requires antibacterial treatment of the axillary area with soap and water, and even with local antibiotics. Shaving the axillary area is also helpful because sweat trapped by hair merely adds to the problem.

Although the apocrine glands reflect our primitive origin, the eccrine glands constitute an advanced, uniquely human system of temperature control. There are several million of these glands scattered over the body surface, with the greatest concentration on the palms, soles, and forehead. Each eccrine gland consists of a coiled tube of cells located in the dermis. These cells secrete a dilute salt solution, which passes through a tunnel traversing the epidermis and then empties through a pore onto the surface of the skin.

When the body becomes overheated, a very small increase in the temperature of the blood will deliver this information to a control center in the brain. A message from the control center travels through the nervous system and activates the eccrine sweat glands. The evaporation of the sweat produced by millions of these glands cools the body, dissipating heat that has been generated either from physical activity or from a high environmental temperature. As the body temperature returns to normal, the brain center sends out messages to the sweat glands, advising them to discontinue their activity.

Perspiration in response to vigorous physical activity can lead to the loss of a large amount of water, to say nothing of the salt that goes along with it. It is estimated that the body can perspire at the rate of two to three quarts of sweat per hour. A day of hard physical labor in a hot environment can easily result in a loss of ten or fifteen quarts of eccrine sweat. Fortunately, the thirst mechanism tells the person to replace the lost water before symptoms of dehydration develop. Salt loss, however, can be another matter, and stomach cramps are often the first warning that salt must be replaced along with the lost water.

If the excessive amounts of water lost through sweating are not replaced, the resultant state of dehydration will reduce the ability to continue to sweat. If there is continued physical activity, then heat stroke, or *hyperthermia*, may occur. In this condition sweating stops completely and the body temperature soars, rising uncontrollably to 105 degrees and sometimes higher. Hyperthermia can cause serious and permanent damage to the brain.

Anybody who has ever sat in a dentist's chair is aware that emotional factors can activate the sweat glands as effectively as a two-mile run. The eccrine glands found on the palms and soles, forehead, and axillary area are particularly sensitive to emotional stimulation. In some individuals, sweating may be inappropriate and excessive, a condition referred to as *hyperhidrosis*. This condition has its psychosomatic overtones (see chapter 15).

BLOOD VESSELS

The extensive network of blood vessels in the dermis complements the sweat glands in controlling body temperature. When the environmental temperature is high or heat is generated through exertion, small blood vessels dilate and more blood passes close to the skin surface, transferring heat outside the body. In contrast, when the external temperature falls and the body is cold, the blood vessels contract, decreasing the blood supply at the surface and thereby conserving body heat. Like the eccrine sweat glands, the superficial blood vessels are also responsive to the emotions. The blood vessels on the face and upper chest are most reactive, and an inappropriate, exaggerated flush or "blush" under stress is a common, albeit sometimes embarrassing, phenomenon.

2 DERMATITIS

The liver can suffer from hepatitis, the kidney from nephritis, and the heart from carditis. The familiar suffix -itis indicates that a state of inflammation exists, but it does not specify the cause. So when your doctor makes a diagnosis of dermatitis, he's indicating that your skin is inflamed but nothing more. The origins of dermatitis are remarkably varied and include allergies, simple irritations, infections, and hereditary defects. To make matters more complicated, there are several distinctive forms of dermatitis of which the causes are unknown.

But the skin changes that occur in all forms of dermatitis are the same, regardless of cause. They are familiar to anyone who has ever changed a diaper or suffered the agonies of poison ivy. The earliest change to take place is redness of the skin (erythema) caused by engorgement and dilation of the small blood vessels. Erythema is usually accompanied by swelling (edema), the result of fluid leaving the damaged blood vessels and accumulating in the tissue. If this swelling is severe, the skin cells of the epidermis are torn apart, forming blisters that fill up with the edema fluid. When the blisters break, the skin "weeps." In some chronic forms of dermatitis, injury to the skin may be protracted but not severe enough to cause a blistering reaction. The distinctive changes in this form of dermatitis are redness, scaling, and thickening of the skin.

IRRITANT CONTACT DERMATITIS

Soap, detergents, ammonia, and the many other powerful cleaning materials that fill the shelves of supermarkets are potential causes of an itchy, at times blistering and at other times dry and cracking rash on the fingers and hands. This condition is so common among homemakers that it has sometimes been called "housewife's eczema."

Homemakers are not the only ones who fall victim to hand rashes from irritating chemicals, however. Doctors and dentists, restaurant workers, bartenders, bricklayers, and a host of industrial workers are among those who suffer from the same disease, caused by a variety of irritants. The common characteristic of these irritating chemicals is that they alter the normal, slightly acidic character of the skin's surface, dissolve its protective oil coating, and/or interfere with the barrier functions of the keratin (top layer) of the skin.

Since the cause of irritant contact hand dermatitis is usually obvious to both doctor and patient, it would seem that a cure should be easy. But it's difficult to expect a mother not to bathe her baby, change the diapers, make a salad, or wash her hair. Try to tell a painter to avoid turpentine, or a bricklayer to go easy on the cement.

If avoidance of the irritating material is not always practical, then protection becomes the next best therapeutic approach. Homemakers with irritant dermatitis should wear cotton gloves under rubber gloves for all "wet" work. (The cotton gloves absorb sweat, another potential irritant.) Alkaline soap should be replaced with a soap substitute, or a soap-and-oil cleansing bar. A protective and lubricating hand cream should be applied during the day, especially after hand washing and after removing the rubber gloves.

Industrial workers with an occupational hand rash may find it impractical to work with rubber gloves or some other form of protective hand covering. For them, protective ointments may be preferable—so-called barrier creams that protect the skin from water and water-soluble chemicals as well as oil and chemicals soluble in oil.

DRY SKIN DERMATITIS

A popular dermatological paradox is that the more you bathe, the drier your skin becomes. This is apparent in many areas of the country in the fall and early winter, when heating systems start to operate and the environmental humidity in the home drops precipitously. Too-frequent bathing during this time of year removes the normal oil barrier from the skin surface and permits evaporation of water from the skin into the atmosphere. Atmospheric water usually replenishes the loss, but because environmental humidity is so low, the skin suffers a net loss. The end result is dry skin, a condition called *xerosis* or, more popularly, the "winter itch."

In severe cases of xerosis, a patchy dermatitis develops, particularly on the arms and legs. Xerotic dermatitis may become unpleasantly persistent unless it is recognized and given proper treatment—one that is both simple and risk-free. Bathing should be brief (one minute or so) in comfortably tepid (not hot) water, and using as little soap as possible (even the super-fatted variety). The application of a moisturizing lotion after bathing traps the imbibed water in the skin and prevents its loss into the atmosphere.

Patients often ask their dermatologists what is the best moisturizer available. In 1986 Consumers Union invited a panel of six hundred women to evaluate and rank forty-eight different moisturizers. The list included a broad spectrum of products ranging from elegant cosmetics that sell for as much as $6.10 per ounce to humble store-brand lotions at $.10 per ounce. The participants in the study did not know the names, cost, or ingredients of the products they were testing. The panel's selections revealed that cost per ounce had little to do with moisturizer performance and user acceptance. In fact, many of the less expensive lotions were rated higher than the more exorbitantly priced cosmetics. The implied conclusion: Don't be fooled by advertising claims, fancy names, or expensive additives. Select a moisturizer that feels comfortable and does the job for you and, above all, don't worry if it's only $2 for the large-size bottle.

Many of the moisturizers on the market today contain urea, a chemical that may be irritating to some but does effectively bind water to the skin. Bath oils and special soaps can also be helpful in treating xerosis and xerotic dermatitis. If the rash associated with xerosis does not respond to simple moisturizers, dermatologists are likely to supplement therapy with a mild, topical corticosteroid in a lubricating cream that will reduce itching and speed up the resolution of the dermatitis.

SEBORRHEIC DERMATITIS

Those embarrassing white flakes that fall from an itchy scalp are the most common signs of *seborrheic dermatitis,* an inflammation of the scalp that at times can affect other areas of the body (eyebrows, face, underarms, chest, upper back, and groin).

Simple dry scalp (some itching and scaling but no inflammation) is best treated with a lubricating (emollient) lotion and a mild, possibly soapless, shampoo. In mild seborrheic dermatitis, you can control the flaking and itching by using one of the over-the-counter shampoos that contain sulfur, salicylic acid, tar derivatives, selenium sulfide, or zinc pyrithione.

But when the dermatitis progresses to red, scaly patches or thick crusting on the scalp or on the body, see your dermatologist. In addition to the over-the-counter products, your doctor can prescribe more potent prescription shampoos. The seborrheic rash in other areas of the body usually responds to salves containing corticosteroids, sulfur, salicylic acid, and antibiotics.

To date, no scientific studies have shown that changes in the diet, or the addition of vitamins or minerals, can control dandruff. Nor is there any evidence to suggest that dandruff may lead to baldness. Although severe dandruff and male-pattern baldness (beginning at the temples and progressing to form a "widow's peak") may occur simultaneously, no cause-and-effect relationship between the two has ever been proven. In fact, dandruff can last for years without leading to the slightest thinning of the hair.

Unfortunately, the cause of seborrheic dermatitis is not

known, and there is no cure for this common disease. However, you can control its most visible and annoying symptoms by using medicated shampoos and other topical medications.

STASIS DERMATITIS

Dermatitis on the lower portion of the legs is often attributable to poor circulation. The presence of varicose veins, attacks of *thrombophlebitis* (an inflammation of the lining of the veins), and obesity are factors that interfere with the flow of blood—against the forces of gravity—from the legs to the heart. Varicose veins have defective valves that are unable to prevent a backflow of blood. The veins stand out, dilated and twisted cords, incapable of moving the blood along in a proper fashion. This sluggish circulation interferes with the normal skin metabolism and *stasis dermatitis* develops in the nutritionally deprived skin.

The earliest signs of impending skin disease are swelling of the ankles and pinpoint brownish discolorations of the skin that occur when the defective blood flow forces red blood cells out of the small skin capillaries. This phenomenon of bleeding into the skin is called *purpura*, and can be a symptom of many diseases of the blood vessels or of the blood-clotting mechanism.

If the stasis circulatory problem persists, a red, itchy dermatitis will appear on the ankles. After years of these intermittent episodes of dermatitis, the rash becomes persistent and the skin unalterably thickened, scarred, and discolored.

Skin ulcers are the most distressing complication of stasis dermatitis. These are painful openings that occur where the full thickness of the skin has been destroyed by a combination of blood vessel disease, injury, and infection. These stasis ulcers are slow to heal and have a tendency to recur following the most minor injury, or even spontaneously.

Preventive measures are the first line of treatment. Elastic bandages or support stockings are invaluable in forestalling dermatitis and leg ulcers in those who suffer from varicose veins. Rest, elevation of the legs while sitting or lying down, and avoidance of prolonged standing are also helpful. For years medical authorities have debated the virtues of destroying varicose veins by injecting them with a chemical that irritates the lining of the vein (sclerotherapy) or removing them surgically. Destruction of the veins or surgery is unlikely to help stasis dermatitis unless it is performed in the early stages of the disease, before the changes in the skin have become persistent and ulcers have appeared.

An acute flare-up of stasis dermatitis calls for very gentle treatment, since the inflamed skin can be sensitive even to rather innocuous, usually well-tolerated local medications. If treatment causes additional irritation, not only will the stasis dermatitis become worse, but an intensely itchy rash may spread rapidly over the entire body. This phenomenon is called *autosensitization*, a term that implies allergy to one's own tissue.

ATOPIC DERMATITIS (ECZEMA)

The word *eczema* is derived from a Greek word meaning "to boil out"—an apt description of the appearance of the skin with severe dermatitis. Eczema, without a qualifying adjective, is sometimes considered synonymous with other forms of dermatitis, an erroneous assumption. Most doctors today quite properly reserve the term *eczema* for the specific, hereditary disease known as *atopic dermatitis*.

The word *atopy* originates from another Greek word, *atopos*, "away from the place." The concept of atopy was introduced in the 1920s to describe a group of familial diseases—hay fever, asthma, and atopic dermatitis—that were considered to be "out of place" in that they were allergic reactions to rather ordinary things such as pollen, dust, and common foods.

For many years, atopic dermatitis was considered to be purely an allergic disease similar in cause to its hereditary companions, asthma and hay fever. This misconception encouraged the use of traditional therapy, an attempt to desensitize the patient with injections or to eliminate the foods and inhaled materials that were thought to produce the symptoms. This approach has not been successful and it is now apparent that the origins of atopic dermatitis are far more complex than the old concepts of allergy could possibly explain.

Atopic dermatitis first appears in infancy. The familiar redness and chapping on a baby's cheeks can be the earliest sign of the disease. Later, dermatitis inflames the skin on the back of the arms and the front of the legs, and subsequently shifts to involve the skin in the folds of the elbows and knees. The rash, in these typical areas, may come and go throughout life although there is a tendency for improvement with advancing age. For most adults, recurrent outbreaks of eczema are a thing of the past.

Common Characteristics of Eczema

Atopic dermatitis is often a question of degree, and can vary in severity from a red blistering rash to a low-grade thickening and discoloration of the skin. It is often impossible to explain why a flare-up occurs or, for that matter, why the rash occasionally disappears. Because an understanding of the fundamental cause of atopic dermatitis is lacking, there is no cure and the treatments offered by dermatologists and allergists are only "symptomatic"—that is, they control only the symptoms. But any treatment program, even a symptomatic one, must take into consideration the following factors:

1. Itchy Skin Itching is hardly a unique symptom. Most forms of dermatitis itch, but few itch with the intensity of atopic dermatitis. Paroxysms of itching may be triggered by such inconsequential stimuli as dressing or undressing, minor changes in temperature, contact with wool or animal fur, or physical activity that induces sweating. The itching sensation demands scratching and initiates the itch-scratch cycle: the more you itch, the more you scratch; the more you scratch, the more you itch. Unlike other chronic skin diseases, the scratching and rubbing in atopic dermatitis causes a thickening of the skin. The abnormally thickened skin sends out more messages of itch, thus fueling a more destructive itch-scratch cycle.

Elimination of the intense and unpredictable itching would go a long way in moderating the disease, but medical science has yet to develop a totally effective and safe anti-itch medication.

2. *Dry Skin* Dry skin is usually an inherited skin abnormality seen in individuals with atopic dermatitis. Often the parents or siblings of the patient with this ailment will also have inherited the dry skin, if not the dermatitis. Since dry skin increases itching, it is important that the atopic individual keep "well oiled" with moisturizing lotions and other emollients, particularly during the winter when skin dryness is at its worst.

Many patients with atopic dermatitis also suffer from a condition called *keratosis pilaris*, a fine bumpy rash on the thighs and upper arms. This condition, determined by heredity, occurs in the relatives of patients with atopic dermatitis and in some nonatopic families as well.

3. *Allergy* Food allergies are no longer considered a major cause of atopic dermatitis. The process of skin testing in order to detect the presence of an allergy to certain foods has proven to be of little value, since the skin tends to respond in an inconsistent manner to the injection of the test materials. Similarly, diet modification as a treatment for atopic dermatitis has not met with much success. Not only are special diets hard on the patient, but the results are difficult to evaluate and probably useless.

As a result, patients with atopic dermatitis should discard those traditional food prejudices that are handed down from generation to generation against such "bad" foods as milk, tomatoes, chocolate, berries, and nuts. It's unreasonable, too, to believe that foods can cause a flare-up of the dermatitis one day but be consumed with impunity a week later. If there is a consistent pattern of a flare-up following the ingestion of a specific food, eliminate that food from the diet, but only on a trial basis. In older children and adults, inhalant allergens may appear to be a more important factor in the cause of atopic dermatitis than food allergies. Atopic dermatitis often becomes worse during the ragweed pollen season or in the spring, when trees and grasses are blooming. In severe cases of atopic dermatitis, an attempt should be made by the patient and the family to eliminate dust, feathers, wool, and animals from the home environment.

4. Skin Infections While it's known that children with atopic dermatitis are prone to certain other forms of allergy, they are also often deficient in the helpful, allergic (immune) response to some infections. Bacterial and viral infections thus frequently complicate atopic dermatitis in some youngsters. This lack of immunity means that, for instance, the practice of vaccinating against smallpox (which has actually been abandoned in many parts of the world because the risk of vaccination far outweighs the chances of contracting this now-rare disease) should not be performed on children with active atopic dermatitis. The virus present in the smallpox vaccine can cause a generalized infection of the skin. Similarly, the herpes simplex virus (the cause of cold sores and fever blisters) can also produce a severe widespread skin infection when atopic dermatitis is in an active phase.

Bacterial skin infections that cause boils and impetigo (see chapter 9) occur with unusual frequency in patients with atopic dermatitis. Antibiotics such as erythromycin or penicillin are necessary to control these infections.

5. Emotional Factors The author participated in a study in which a group of patients with severe, intractable atopic dermatitis—patients for whom all other forms of treatment had failed—were treated with psychotherapy and *no other medications*. A statistically significant number of these patients experienced improvement in their dermatitis, only to relapse weeks to months later, after the psychotherapy was discontinued.

Of course, one can argue the question of precedence: Do emotional problems trigger dermatitis in those individuals already predisposed by heredity to get the disorder, or do patients with a chronic and severe skin problem develop emotional symptoms that have an adverse effect on their skin disease?

Many patients with atopic dermatitis do show signs of anger and depression, and some psychiatrists believe that the rash has its beginnings in these emotions. They postulate that inappropriate hostility in these people has turned inward, and scratch-

21

ing becomes a self-destructive method of releasing anger. Other specialists perceive the problem from a different perspective, asking: Why shouldn't the individual with atopic dermatitis be angry and depressed, when he or she is constantly suffering from an uncomfortable, disfiguring, and incapacitating disease?

In this ongoing controversy, everyone can agree that, as with most chronic diseases, patients with severe atopic dermatitis need the emotional support of their family, friends, and physicians to help alleviate the mental anguish of the malady. The rules for care and treatment of atopic dermatitis are not hard-and-fast, but they should include certain guidelines:

1. Protect the skin from irritating and itch-provoking substances such as wool, synthetic fibers, animal fur, and soap.
2. Keep the skin well lubricated, but *not* with excessively greasy substances that block the sweat pores and increase itching.
3. Be realistic about the role of allergy in this disease. Let your observations and not your prejudices be your guide.
4. Use medications prescribed by your doctor to relieve itching and diminish inflammation of the skin.
5. Check frequently for possible infectious complications and be sure that they are treated promptly.

Another form of dermatitis, *allergic contact dermatitis*, results when the skin comes into contact with an allergenic substance, such as poison ivy (see page 52).

DERMATITIS: A GENERAL GUIDE TO TREATMENT

Certain principles apply to the treatment of *all* forms of dermatitis, regardless of the cause, including the acute blistering dermatitis on one hand, or chronic, dry, thick-skinned dermatitis on the other. A well-known dermatologic dictum states: "If the skin is wet, then bathe it, but if it is dry, don't wet it."

This apparent contradiction can be explained in part by the fact that bathing or compressing an area of oozing dermatitis not only soothes but also cleanses the skin, softens and ruptures blisters, and causes drying through evaporation of the compress solution. However, bathing the dry, scaly form of dermatitis removes the protective skin oils that enhance water evaporation. As a result, the inflamed skin becomes even drier and itching may increase.

Wet Dressings

When treating a "weeping" skin rash, apply a wet dressing intermittently. A typical schedule includes the application of a compress three or four times a day for fifteen minutes. Continuous or prolonged bathing of the area would cause the skin to become waterlogged and soggy.

It may come as a surprise to most people that the various chemicals dissolved in water to be used for a compress (or a therapeutic bath) have little to do with the actual value of this procedure. It has long been part of the mystique of the treatment to recommend that small amounts of epsom salts, table salt, or boric acid be dissolved in large quantities of water. This homeopathic approach eliminates any potential problem of toxicity from these chemicals, but it also negates any therapeutic value of the acid or salt used in the solution, since they are used in such small quantities as to be almost useless.

There are several materials used in compress solutions that do have some therapeutic clout. The dermatologist can prescribe potassium permanganate (one grain in one quart of water), which is, at the very least, a good deodorizer and may produce some antibacterial action as well. It is, however, difficult to prepare and it stains everything a deep purple, including skin, nails, or the bathroom rug. Aluminum acetate (Burow's solution) is another old favorite. A concentration of approximately 0.5 percent can be prepared by dissolving a commercially available aluminum acetate tablet or powder in one pint of water. Burow's solution is a very weak antiseptic, but not totally without value. Several other antibiotics can be dissolved in water without destroying their antibacterial effectiveness, but antibiotic solutions are reserved for wet dressings used in treating infected dermatitis.

Most medications that are applied to the skin are made up of one or more active ingredients and a "vehicle." The vehicle facilitates the delivery of the active medication to the ailing skin, and also provides a climate that favors a normal healing process. In the case of compresses or baths, water is both the vehicle and the major active ingredient.

Lotions, Creams, and Ointments

Lotions are another formulation in which water—or sometimes alcohol—is both the vehicle and, to a large extent, the active ingredient. Calamine lotion is an ancient and familiar example; it's composed of water, talc, and several relatively inert metallic oxides, such as zinc oxide. Calamine lotion works in the following manner: When the lotion is applied, the water evaporates and dries the skin; the talc and other ingredients are deposited on the skin surface, producing further drying through absorption. Calamine lotion is also an example of an old-fashioned "shake lotion." Separation of the ingredients occurs when the lotion sits on the shelf, and it is thus necessary to "shake well before using" to resuspend the ingredients in the fluid.

Lotions and liniments (lotions with some oil added) have been replaced by a variety of new vehicle bases—emulsions—created by the pharmaceutical and cosmetic industry. These emulsion bases have revolutionized dermatologic therapy in recent years. An emulsion is a preparation in which an oily substance and water are brought together, mixed completely, and bound at a molecular level by a so-called emulsifying agent. If the emulsion is composed largely of water and only a little of oil, then it has some of the properties of lotion. When this oil-in-water type of emulsion is applied to the skin, the water component will completely evaporate (the familiar vanishing-cream effect), and only a small amount of oil residue will remain on the surface of the skin. Oil-in-water emulsions have drying properties and are generally referred to as creams.

At the other end of the water-oil scale there are emulsions that are composed of a large quantity of an oily material emulsified with only a small amount of water. When this water-in-oil emulsion is broken down on the skin surface, it deposits a thick layer of oil. This produces a lubrication of the skin and a further occlusive effect that blocks the evaporation of water. Emulsion bases that are composed of oil with only small quantities of water are referred to as ointments; they have a greasy tactile sensation. There are currently dozens of emulsion bases with different properties on the market, and new ones appear all the time.

In the treatment of dermatitis, emulsion bases are selected by virtue of their drying or lubricating properties. In the case of a wet dermatitis, apply a medication with a cream base to the skin in between the intermittent wet dressings. This application facilitates further drying, as well as depositing the active medication suspended in the cream on the area of the dermatitis. In a less acute, or drier dermatitis, one might select an in-between type of emulsion base—that is, not too greasy and not too drying.

For the chronic, very dry, and scaly dermatitis, choose an ointment-type emulsion: lots of oil and only a little water. Such a base would have a lubricating effect and therefore trap water in the dry, inflamed skin. The natural counterpart of an ointment-type emulsion is petrolatum (petroleum jelly), which is composed of a mixture of materials obtained from petroleum.

Antibiotics

There are literally dozens of active medications that can be suspended in an appropriate vehicle for the treatment of dermatitis. The two categories of medications that outsell all others put together are the antibiotics and the corticosteroids. Topical antibiotics are often prescribed in treating all forms of dermatitis because infection is a frequent complication that develops even before the patient seeks medical attention. Raw, wet, inflamed skin is the natural habitat of all sorts of germs commonly found in the environment.

The choice of an antibiotic to be applied to the skin is determined by several factors. Since the application of a foreign substance to inflamed skin is certainly one of the most effective ways of creating an allergy, antibiotics that are weak allergy producers are always selected by physicians for topical use. This eliminates penicillin, streptomycin, and the sulfa drugs from consideration. Your doctor would also select an antibiotic that is not used to treat more serious internal infections, since you could experience serious internal allergic reactions by taking a medication that initially caused an allergic rash on your skin. (And you also could not use this antibiotic again, even for a life-threatening illness.)

Fortunately, there are a number of antibiotics that fit the necessary criteria for topical use. Preparations containing bacitracin, gentamicin, polymyxin, and gramicidin are available singly and in combinations. Neomycin is a very effective and widely used antibiotic, but it is a relatively common cause of allergic sensitization, far exceeding that of the other antibiotics mentioned above. In fact, when allergic dermatitis develops during the use of a multiple-antibiotic ointment, it is usually due to the presence of neomycin in the preparation.

Corticosteroids

The use of corticosteroids, both topically and systemically, has changed dermatologic therapy radically since this group of drugs appeared on the market in the 1950s. *Corticosteroids* are drugs that are chemically and functionally similar to natural cortisone produced by the adrenal glands, and they are effective in the treatment of many different skin diseases. They are relatively safe *if used properly*, a fact not appreciated by most patients and many physicians.

It all started with hydrocortisone, the first steroid (short for corticosteroid) to be used topically. Over the years, research chemists have manipulated the basic steroid chemical structure in an effort to increase the drug's therapeutic effectiveness and decrease its undesirable side effects. Their efforts have been particularly successful as far as enhancing the strength of these drugs, and there are currently available a number of very potent topical steroids.

Sales of steroid preparations for use on the skin amount to millions of dollars yearly and the market continues to expand.

Almost annually, new and allegedly better formulations appear on the scene to claim their share of the market. The competition and infighting in the pharmaceutical industry for a share of the steroid market is fierce—a case of pharmaceutical overkill in which research and advertising dollars are being wasted to out-steroid the competition. (The result is that the consumer has to pay more for the product.)

Regardless of the cause, inflammation of the skin due to dermatitis can be diminished by corticosteroid preparations. They are especially useful in irritant contact dermatitis, allergic contact dermatitis (see page 52), atopic dermatitis, and seborrheic dermatitis. Symptomatically, they relieve itching and reduce the scratch-related complications of these diseases. They also can be used safely with undiminished potency in combination with other drugs, including the topical antibiotics.

A doctor's choice of a specific topical steroid preparation depends upon several factors. Cost and availability are certainly major concerns, but the usual deciding factor is the strength of the preparation, which is inversely related to its safety. Topical steroids fall into three general categories—high potency, mid potency, and low potency—and there are in-between categories as well. As a general rule the most potent steroids are used for short-term treatment on limited areas of the body, while the milder steroids are used for more protracted therapy, often on large areas of skin.

Side effects from the topical corticosteroids are relatively uncommon, considering how much they are used. The long-term use of the strongest steroids on certain areas of the body where absorption into the skin is great (under the arms, in the groin area, and on the face) can cause changes that usually are irreversible when the medication is discontinued. Thinning of the skin and underlying connective tissue can lead to the appearance of stretch marks, and small, permanently dilated blood vessels may appear on the surface of the steroid-thinned skin. This steroid-weakened skin is very sensitive to bruising, and black-and-blue marks appear from mild or even unnoticed trauma.

These complications can be minimized by using only hydrocortisone or one of its low-potency variants on skin that is likely to develop changes from the more potent steroids. Hydrocortisone, although not as effective as the newer steroids, will rarely weaken the skin by thinning out the connective tissue. Still, many forms of dermatitis of any significance must be treated with stronger topical steroids. Limiting the frequency and duration of their use will usually prevent thinning of the skin.

Another possible complication of topical corticosteroid use must be considered when large areas of the body are being treated for prolonged periods. Under these circumstances, steroids can be absorbed into the body in quantities sufficient to produce general systemic side effects, a major one being the inhibition of the adrenal gland's normal production of cortisone-like substances. Fortunately for the public, potent topical corticosteroids are available only through prescription. It is the responsibility of the physician, as well as the sensible patient, to limit the use of these drugs to prevent serious side effects.

Systemic Medications

Systemic medications are drugs that are taken internally rather than applied topically, and they include the counterparts of the topical medications already mentioned. Systemic antibiotics play a role when an infection is too extensive or deep in the skin for one to rely on topical antibiotics alone. Systemic corticosteroids are also useful in severe forms of allergic contact dermatitis, since they can be discontinued after a brief and finite period of therapy. Medical judgment dictates whether these drugs should be used in other more persistent forms of dermatitis. Consideration should always be given to the fact that while corticosteroids suppress the inflammation and allergic reaction of dermatitis, they do not eliminate its cause. Because of this, protracted use of the drug in many skin diseases becomes inevitable and, unfortunately, patients occasionally become "hooked" on corticosteroids since they relieve the symptoms of dermatitis like no other form of therapy presently available.

Systemic medications are also often prescribed to relieve the intense itching associated with many forms of dermatitis. The itching sensation is believed to be transmitted by the same nerve fibers that carry the sensation of pain. In fact, the almost instinctive scratch response may be a means of substituting mild pain for itch—pain in this case may prove to be a more tolerable sensation. Because a formula for an effective anti-itch medication has yet to reach the drawing board, the antihistamines are the most widely prescribed group of drugs for this symptom. They appear to be effective when given in doses that are high enough to cause sedation. Many of them, however, seem to be only a little bit better than ordinary aspirin, which has anti-itch as well as analgesic properties. Several tranquilizers have been developed specifically for the treatment of itching but, like the antihistamines, they are most effective when they cause sedation.

HOME TREATMENT

There are some forms of treatment that you can do yourself to relieve minor symptoms of dermatitis, once this disorder has been diagnosed by a physician. Check with your doctor to make sure these procedures are suitable for your particular skin problem.

Wet Dermatitis

Treat wet dermatitis with compresses or total body baths. Remember, water is the active ingredient in this type of therapy. Most of the commonly used additives are neither harmful nor particularly helpful, although baking soda or a commercial colloid preparation suspended in the bath water may be useful for temporary relief of severe itching. Between wet dressings, apply a soothing lotion or cream. It will add to the drying effect and bring therapeutic medications into contact with the dermatitis. A physician may prescribe an antibiotic or corticosteroid cream, depending upon the cause or complications of the dermatitis.

Do not overdry the skin. When blistering and exudation (weeping) stop, discontinue all wet dressings.

Dry Dermatitis

Treat dry dermatitis either with emulsion ointments that consist predominantly of oil or with home remedies that have a lubricating effect, such as petrolatum, mineral oil, or even solid vegetable oil. Do not use compresses or overbathe dry, scaly dermatitis; doing so will only increase the dryness and itching.

All Forms of Dermatitis

Always use bland anti-itch lotions. Avoid over-the-counter preparations that contain anesthetics, antihistamines, or other chemicals alleged to relieve itching—they may cause allergic reactions when applied to inflamed skin.

Over-the-counter oral antihistamines, however, may be taken when necessary. Follow the directions on the package as to dosage and precautions. Although not always effective in relieving itching, they are generally safe to use. If dermatitis becomes more severe, discontinue all treatment and reconsult your dermatologist.

3 PSORIASIS

In the United States more than one percent of the population is afflicted with psoriasis, a chronic skin disease that can vary in severity from a few localized eruptions to a widespread, incapacitating body rash. Psoriasis typically starts with a small red papule with a barely perceptible scale. This enlarges into a red patch, often several inches in diameter, that produces silvery white scales that continuously flake off and reform. Although psoriasis can appear anywhere on the body, the common areas affected are the elbows and knees, the scalp, and the genital area.

The cause of psoriasis is not known. It is a hereditary disease controlled by a dominant gene with incomplete expressivity—in other words, one parent carrying the gene can pass the disease on to a child, but the disease may or may not "express" itself during the child's lifetime. What exactly is inherited is unknown, although theories abound. Current favorites include an aberration of the skin's response to injury and inflammation, and abnormal behavior of the cells that regulate immunity.

Not infrequently psoriasis is triggered by an injury to normal-appearing skin. A severe sunburn can evolve into psoriasis in a predisposed person. A surgical incision can become a line of psoriasis, or the friction of a belt or shoe can provoke the disease at the point of irritation. In children a totally unrelated rash, such as chicken pox, can turn into psoriasis and, for unknown reasons, an infection such as a strep throat or any upper respiratory infection can trigger a rash composed of dozens of small spots of psoriasis.

The same disease process that attacks the skin can affect the nails. A buildup of dry scaly material under the nails and the separation of the nail plate from the underlying bed are characteristic changes. A milder form of nail psoriasis creates pits or small depressions that stipple the nail plate.

Some patients with psoriasis also suffer from a form of arthritis that is similar but not identical to rheumatoid arthritis. Like the psoriasis itself, the arthritis can vary from relatively mild intermittent swellings of the fingers and toes, to a severe disabling form of psoriasis of the large joints and spine. The severity of the arthritis does not necessarily parallel the extent of the psoriasis, and the two conditions may be related only in that they reflect the same genetic disease.

Through the efforts of research scientists throughout the world, information has been gathered about the behavior of psoriatic skin that has helped our understanding of some of the traditional methods of treatment. One of the key observations is that the epidermal cells in victims of psoriasis are dividing and keratinizing (changing into scale) far more rapidly than the cells of normal skin. Many of the medicines that have been used successfully against psoriasis over the years have inhibited or slowed down this abnormally rapid process.

TREATMENT OF PSORIASIS

Topical Medications

When psoriasis occurs in limited areas of the skin, the favored therapies are the corticosteroid creams, ointments, gels, and lotions. Since externally applied corticosteroids can have side effects locally as well as internally (thinning of the skin and suppression of the normal adrenal gland function), it is important that the physician select a steroid of the appropriate strength and regulate its usage carefully. For example, there are now extremely powerful corticosteroid preparations that are used for a two-week period, followed by a respite. At the other end of the spectrum are mild steroids that can be applied over large areas for long periods with little risk of side effects.

Small areas of psoriasis also can be treated by injecting a liquid suspension of corticosteroid into the skin, a technique that delivers the medication to the diseased area more efficiently than an ointment applied to the skin surface. Since much of the injected steroid finds its way into the bloodstream, the potential exists for systemic side effects, so the number of injections must be limited.

One of the ancient and traditional treatment methods for psoriasis uses a mixture of chemicals that are by-products of heating coal or its residue, coke, to very high temperatures. The black viscous liquid that is the end stage of this process is called *crude coal tar*, and is used in ointments to treat psoriasis as well as some forms of dermatitis. A synthetic drug, anthralin, similar to tar, is also effective in treating chronic patches of psoriasis. Its drawbacks are that it temporarily discolors the skin and at times is quite irritating.

Phototherapy

Ultraviolet light has been used to treat psoriasis since the beginning of the century—first in the form of natural sunlight and later with artificial light sources. Sometimes a tar ointment is applied to the skin prior to the ultraviolet therapy, a procedure that enhances the effectiveness of the ultraviolet. This form of treatment, called the Goeckerman regimen, is used widely in doctors' offices, hospitals, and psoriasis day-care centers. Although it is not curative, it will clear or significantly improve the skin of many psoriatic patients. Usually a maintenance treatment program must be continued to avoid relapse.

A form of phototherapy similar to the Goeckerman regimen has been widely used for the past ten years. It is called *PUVA*, an acronym for *psoralen*, an oral medication that sensitizes the skin to ultraviolet light, and UVA, the long-wave form of ultraviolet light. The psoralen is ingested two hours before treatment. Then ultraviolet light is carefully administered in increasing exposure times. The results are good, with over 75 percent of patients clearing or experiencing significant improvement after several months of such therapy. Like the Goeckerman treatment, PUVA therapy requires trained personnel supervising the treatments in order to prevent skin burns and other complications. There is still some unresolved concern about the long-term side effects of PUVA, particularly the possibility of inducing skin cancer later in life.

A more natural form of phototherapy can be found at treatment centers in Israel, at the Dead Sea. Since the Dead Sea is the lowest topographical point on the earth's surface, the sunlight reaching patients there has been filtered through the atmosphere, so almost all the harmful rays are gone. This fact, plus exposure to the high mineral content of the Dead Sea, helps to heal many cases of psoriasis. However, the treatment is expensive and time-consuming, and there is no guarantee of a cure.

Internal Medications

Methotrexate and other chemotherapeutic cancer drugs are now used to treat severe, disabling psoriasis. Although these medications can be very effective, they need careful monitoring as they are potentially toxic to other tissues of the body. The liver and the blood cells as well as the cells lining the gastrointestinal tract are particularly sensitive to methotrexate-induced damage. While the response to methotrexate is variable, in many patients it produces remarkable improvement. But, as with most other forms of treatment, if the drug is discontinued the psoriasis generally returns.

Corticosteroids given by pill or injection are effective in clearing psoriasis, but a severe "rebound" flare-up of the condition when the dose is reduced, or the drug discontinued, make this treatment unacceptable except in rare circumstances.

The newest oral medication for psoriasis is *etretinate*, a type of vitamin-A derivative similar in many ways to *isotretinoin* (Accutane), the drug used to treat severe cystic acne. The manufacturer of etretinate recommends its use in only the most severe forms of psoriasis that fail to respond to all the treatments described above, including methotrexate. There is a long list of side effects attributed to this medication, including the development of fetal abnormalities in women who take it during pregnancy. In fact, because etretinate remains in the body for months to years after a course of therapy is completed, it is not a recommended form of treatment for women of childbearing age. Liver damage, bone changes, and an increase in blood lipids are other potentially serious side effects. Despite these possible complications, some rare cases of severe psoriasis may warrant treatment with this new drug.

4 ACNE

Acne is a disorder of the *pilosebaceous unit* of the skin. Each unit consists of a hair follicle and the sebaceous gland attached to it. The sebaceous gland secretes *sebum*, an oily substance, into the follicle and through the follicle pore onto the skin surface.

One cause of acne is a defect in the cells that form the lining of the follicle. They do not mature (keratinize) in a normal fashion, and thus form a blockage of the pore or the follicle itself. The area of blockage is seen on the surface of the skin as a blackhead or whitehead (comedone). But the inflammatory lesions of acne—the papules (pimples), pustules, and acne cysts—are caused by bacteria breaking down the sebum into irritating fatty acids that attract pus cells into and around the follicle.

As we will see, acne can be effectively treated by correcting the defect in the follicle lining cells, destroying the bacteria that act on sebum, or by decreasing the amount of sebum produced by the sebaceous glands.

CAUSES OF ACNE

Although the exact cause of acne is still a mystery, there are clearly a number of factors that, if not decisive, play significant roles in this skin condition.

Genetic Inheritance

Certain inherited characteristics make some young people seem more likely than others to experience acne. The most serious cases occur among youngsters whose parents, either one or both, suffered from severe acne in their youth. Studies have shown that identical twins tend to suffer from acne to an almost identical degree. Although the genetic predisposition is evident, the manner in which these inherited traits express themselves and determine acne susceptibility is not yet clearly understood.

Excessive Skin Oil

Since acne appears in areas of the body that are noted for their large and numerous oil glands, it would be logical to assume that an overproduction of the skin oil sebum is the direct cause of the acne lesion. As a matter of fact, there have been several studies that show a rough correlation between high levels of oil production and the severity of the acne: the more oily the skin, the more numerous the pimples. This simplistic explanation is lacking, however, because there are many young people with oily skin and not a trace of acne, to say nothing of the young adults who experience acne and dry skin at the same time. A conservative conclusion can be drawn: Acne is frequently associated with excessive skin oil, but oily skin is not a prerequisite for acne to develop.

Hormonal Factors

Androgens (male sex hormones) are produced by the testes in males, the ovaries in females, and the adrenal glands in both sexes. These hormones are the most important regulators of the size and activity of the oil glands. At puberty, there is a marked increase in the amount of androgens produced by the sex glands in both males and females, which results in an increase in both the size of the oil glands and the quantity of oil production.

It would be convenient if acne could be explained by the presence of large amounts of androgens in acne-prone youngsters. Unfortunately, this is not the case. Most youngsters with acne, both male and female, produce perfectly normal quantities of androgens for their respective sexes.

Infections

Patients with pustular and cystic forms of acne often erroneously believe that they have a number of skin infections. But acne is not considered an infection in the accepted sense of the word, although there are skin bacteria living and multiplying in the oil glands and ducts that channel sebum to the skin surface, and these undoubtedly play a contributory role in the formation of the acne lesions. Current medical theory suggests that these bacteria do change elements of the skin oil into irritating chemicals that are responsible, in part, for acne inflammation.

Emotional Factors

While bacteria, hormones, and large oil glands are possible causes of acne, is it also possible that acne is primarily a psychosomatic disorder? Can stress lead to a flare-up of pimples and lesions on the skin of a susceptible person? It's difficult to evaluate the role that emotions play in any illness in which a single specific cause has yet to be identified. Acne, more than many other skin disorders, is characterized by periods of active eruption followed by unpredictable periods when the skin remains relatively clear. Many patients choose to believe that acne flare-ups are related to the ordinary stresses of living: work-related problems, school examinations, or interpersonal friction. It is difficult to dispute the fact that there *are* times when anxiety or tension may trigger acne. It is also apparent that some individuals appear to be more susceptible to emotional influences than are others. But the role of emotions in acne is often overemphasized by patients who seem to be searching for some explanation, however tenuous, for the erratic nature of this skin disorder.

There is one aspect of the acne problem in which emotions are of paramount importance, and that is in the almost universal desire to open, pick at, or in some way manipulate existing skin blemishes. In most acne patients, this self-destructive practice is limited to an occasional, ill-advised assault on a few very unsightly pimples. The motivation is reasonable: to eliminate the blemish more rapidly instead of waiting through the seeming eternity of the normal healing process. But in some, the desire is excessive and self-defeating, since the end result of picking—scars and disfigurement—far exceeds the acne blemishes as a cosmetic problem.

In some instances, though, "picking" becomes a form of compulsive behavior. A quick look in a mirror will trigger a session of picking and squeezing. After the episode the patient may feel remorse, but more self-destructive episodes usually follow.

Since this self-mutilation can be caused by emotional disturbances of varying degrees, each patient's problem must be handled individually. Most acne sufferers respond to a physician's explanation of the negative effects of picking the skin and welcome suitable forms of alternative therapy. But sometimes the self-mutilation is more severe, and some patients become angry at the very suggestion that they are damaging their own skin. Sometimes psychiatric help may be needed to overcome the compulsion; ideally, however, the patient should come to this conclusion on his or her own.

Diet

Traditionally, parents have believed that dietary abuse was the major cause of acne in teenagers. "If you would only stop eating all that junk . . . ," has been a cry heard in homes throughout the land. Physicians have gone along with diet modifications, and at various times singled out chocolate, cola drinks, sugar, greasy foods, iodine, and "acid" as contributing to the acne problem.

It is understandable that acne sufferers would focus on their dietary indiscretions to explain the otherwise inexplicable off-and-on-again behavior of acne blemishes. But a number of scientific studies tend to contradict this assumption. One of the most interesting investigations sought to evaluate the effects of large amounts of chocolate on patients with active acne. One half of a group of volunteers was given large chocolate bars daily, while the other group received a chocolate substitute that was indistinguishable from the real thing. When the study was completed, the two groups were carefully examined and there was no difference in the acne in either group of volunteers. Other foods have been similarly studied, and discarded, as possible aggravators of acne.

TREATMENT

Despite the continuing confusion concerning the causes of acne, there have been several worthwhile advances in its treatment. Of course, no single medication able to effect a total cure is presently available, or likely to become so in the near future. Every patient under treatment for the problem should be aware that almost all of the current forms of therapy merely control acne symptoms. For many people, the withdrawal of treatment may trigger a relapse; others may "outgrow" the condition entirely.

People with mild cases of acne can probably control their problem with the judicious use of some over-the-counter medications, plus gentle cleansing of the affected area, and avoidance of picking and squeezing of blackheads or pimples. (For more severe cases, see your dermatologist.) The following forms of treatment can help a great deal in modifying or eliminating the worst aspects of this distressing condition.

Topical Medications

Although personal hygiene has little to do with the production of comedones and acne lesions, frequent but gentle washing with medicated soaps or detergents continues to be a form of treatment advocated by some but not all doctors. More profound drying and peeling of facial acne can be accomplished with some of the traditional sulfur and salicylic acid lotions as well as two other chemicals, benzoyl peroxide, the mainstay of many over-the-counter best sellers, and tretinoin, a prescription medication.

Benzoyl peroxide, in lotion, cream, or gel form, or incorporated in a cleansing bar, not only dries the skin and promotes peeling but penetrates the oil ducts, where it kills the bacteria that break down sebum into acne-producing fatty acids. Tretinoin, sold only by prescription as a cream, lotion, or gel, also dries and peels the skin. But its primary therapeutic function is to normalize the epidermal cells around the old duct openings, thus eliminating the comedones. Excessive drying and peeling of the skin can be reduced by using a mild concentration of tretinoin or by reducing the frequency of application.

Abrasive therapy—cleansing bars or creams containing particulate abradants or specially designed abrasive sponges—is of little value in clearing up acne. These mechanical cleansers, moreover, can be irritating to the skin, especially when they are used in combination with other topical medications.

Unfortunately, excessive drying of the skin resulting in a red, scaly rash is a common side reaction of most topical medications. This problem should not be treated with dry-skin creams, which only block up more of the oil duct pores and aggravate the condition. While there are moisturizers on the market that are purported to be "noncomedogenic" (they don't block up pores), it's preferable to discontinue all external treatment and to resume it on a more limited basis only when the dryness, redness, and flaking have abated.

Women afflicted with acne are naturally interested in selecting cosmetics that will be compatible with treatment, or at least won't exacerbate the existing condition. In general, water-based makeups are well tolerated by the disturbed skin, while oil-based cosmetics tend to clog pores and encourage the formation of more comedones. Some of the over-the-counter medications available for acne sufferers are prepared as skin-tinted lotions and can be used as a makeup foundation. Still, they may not be as effective from the cosmetic standpoint as are oil-free cosmetics.

Ultraviolet Light, X Rays, and the Fast Freeze

The therapeutic value of sunlight for various skin conditions has been recognized since ancient times. Little more than seventy-five years ago, heliotherapy (sun treatment) was used to treat skin infections, including tuberculosis of the skin. Ultraviolet light, in the form of natural sunlight or a commercial sunlamp, produces redness, peeling, and often a tanning of the skin. Tanning often brings a much-welcome cosmetic improvement.

There are those who dispute the proposition that ultraviolet light clears up acne. Moreover, many acne patients experience a flare-up of their skin problem in the summer or following a vacation in a sunny environment. But the fact remains that most youngsters with acne do well over the summer and may not need to return for treatment until October and November. A more serious argument against ultraviolet light has come with increasing knowledge of its long-term harmful effects on the skin. Therefore, exposure to the sun or artificial ultraviolet light should not be prescribed as a form of acne therapy.

Yet another favorite technique frequently used by dermatologists in their offices is to quick-freeze the skin with "slush" (a mixture of dry ice and acetone), or with super-cold liquid nitrogen. The redness and peeling that ensue provide, at the very least, a brief cosmetic improvement in the skin.

Superficial X ray, once a very popular form of therapy, is rarely used these days because of a legitimate concern with the long-term effects of radiation on the skin. In the past, excessive amounts of X-ray therapy for acne led to skin changes that made the treated area susceptible to the development of skin cancers many years after the therapy was completed. Furthermore, there is real concern about the possibility of thyroid cancer developing in patients who were treated with X ray years ago. Many were not properly protected, and they may have received radiation to the vulnerable area on the front of the neck.

If correctly used, X-ray treatments do shrink the oil glands and cause an impressive but temporary improvement in severe cases of acne. The availability of other forms of effective treatment, however, as well as the long-term consequences of X rays, have turned most doctors and their patients away from this therapeutic modality.

Antibiotics

An important breakthrough in the modern treatment of acne occurred in the 1950s when it was noted that certain antibiotics, particularly tetracycline, were extremely helpful in controlling the symptoms of acne. Antibiotics kill bacteria living in the oil ducts that contribute to the formation of acne blemishes. Today dermatologists often begin their treatment with the conventional amounts of tetracycline that are used to treat infectious diseases, then usually reduce the dose to a fraction of this amount, which still controls the acne. These antibiotics, of course, are available only by prescription.

Many parents of youngsters on long-term tetracycline therapy, a period ranging from months to years, have been realistically skeptical about the safety of this medication. But the years of experience with the drug and the administration of millions of doses in the treatment of acne have proven that tetracycline is both safe and effective. Tetracycline is not without potential side effects, but most of these are mild and disappear quite promptly when the medication is discontinued. Symptoms related to the gastrointestinal tract, including constipation and diarrhea, are among the most common complaints. Sometimes, too, the patient can experience difficulty in swallowing if the tetracycline capsule irritates the lining of the esophagus.

Young women on tetracycline are also subject to a vaginal infection caused by a fungus called *Candida albicans*. This occurs when the antibiotic destroys the normal bacteria that live in the lower intestine. The fungi that are normally kept in check by these bacteria are able to increase in number, leave the intestine, and infect the skin and the vagina. This complication subsides if the tetracycline is discontinued and an appropriate antifungal medication is prescribed (see chapter 9).

Tetracycline cannot be prescribed for pregnant women since it interferes with normal bone and tooth development in the fetus. And young children who take tetracycline for prolonged periods can show a yellowish discoloration of the teeth. This complication, however, does not occur after bone and tooth growth is complete.

Except for increased sensitivity to sunburn, skin reactions to tetracycline are quite rare. Patients who are taking tetracycline during the summer months and who might spend time at the beach should be aware that they may develop a severe, vacation-ending burn after relatively minimal amounts of sun exposure. It's best to stop taking tetracycline a few days before sun exposure and not to resume taking the drug until those days in the sun are over.

For reasons that are not entirely clear, tetracycline may lose its therapeutic effectiveness after months of usage. When this happens, the patient and doctor will notice many new acne lesions forming even though increased doses of tetracycline do not stop the outbreak. The patient may then be advised to switch to another antibiotic, such as erythromycin, which is chemically quite different from tetracycline. Sometimes, more costly tetracycline derivatives such as minocycline, doxycycline, or demeclocycline will do the job when tetracycline has lost its effectiveness or when it fails to work well in the beginning of treatment.

For good reason, most people have an aversion to taking systemic medication in the form of oral antibiotics. This is particularly true when a course of treatment is measured in months or years. But a recent therapeutic development now appears to be a happy compromise for those who are reluctant to embark upon long-term treatment with oral antibiotics. Certain antibiotics in pill form can be dissolved in alcohol and gels without destroying their potency. When applied directly on the skin, these antibiotic solutions penetrate the follicles and deliver medication to the acne blemishes. Although these topical antibiotic preparations are not quite as effective as their systemic counterparts, they seldom cause internal side effects either.

One of the most popular antibiotics that can be used topically is clindamycin, which stops acne breakouts when taken orally but may cause severe irritation of the lower intestine. This potentially serious side effect makes it a risky choice as an oral treatment for acne. On the other hand, clindamycin works well when applied to the skin, and since only very small amounts are absorbed into the body, intestinal irritation and other unpleasant reactions are unlikely. Other similar topical preparations contain tetracycline or erythromycin as the active ingredient. A topical antibiotic used in conjunction with tretinoin or benzoyl peroxide (or sometimes all three) is an effective approach to controlling most cases of mild to moderately severe acne.

Hormones

Two types of hormones are used to treat severe acne when antibiotics fail to stop pustules and cysts from forming. The corticosteroid hormones are very useful in this regard, and can be justifiably prescribed for a short period of time when scarring seems a likely result of acne. Corticosteroids can create havoc with many of the body's normal functions, and should be used only as a stopgap measure. The injection of a small amount of a corticosteroid solution into individual, persistent acne cysts, however, is a safe, effective technique that shrinks the lesion and helps avoid further inflammation and scarring.

By chance more than design, birth control pills have helped acne problems in many women. Estrogen is the active ingredient in the combination pill that can decrease the size and activity of the oil glands. Usually the amount of estrogen necessary to do this is too great to be generally used, except in the most resistant of cases. Moreover, the number of women being treated for acne with large-dose estrogen therapy has decreased dramatically since the advent of Accutane.

Furthermore, a relapse of the acne is common after treatment with birth control pills is discontinued. In fact, the birth control pill has bred a new form of acne. Many women have developed acne for the first time in their lives after discontinuing the pill. Once it occurs, this rebound form of acne may take many months to subside.

The major objections to taking estrogens for acne are the same ones raised in evaluating its use in the pill as a method of birth control. Minor side effects include nausea, weight gain, and emotional upsets, but more serious potential problems can involve the heart, liver, and blood vessels. Dermatologists also see their share of pill-induced complaints, including disturbances of skin pigmentation, hair loss, and an increased susceptibility to vaginal fungus infection.

Isotretinoin (Accutane)

This vitamin A–like compound is a potent and effective drug for the treatment of cystic acne, but it's reserved for the most serious, intractable cases because of its many possible side effects. The long list includes minor problems such as dry skin, chapped lips, eye irritation, nosebleeds, and temporary hair loss, to much more serious problems such as liver function abnormalities, elevation of the lipids in the blood, headaches, and bone problems. The most serious side effect of Accutane, however, is the occurrence of birth defects in babies whose mothers took the drug during pregnancy. For that reason, and because women often do not know they are pregnant during the first weeks or months of gestation, birth control is mandatory when using the drug. Effective contraception must be used for at least one month before the start of Accutane therapy, during therapy, and for one month following the end of therapy. It is recommended that two reliable forms of contraception be used simultaneously (unless abstinence is the chosen method). Careful monitoring of the patient by the doctor and periodic blood tests are also essential during treatment with isotretinoin.

Isotretinoin is administered as a four-to-five-month course of treatment. Improvement in the skin is gradual, and a flare-up of the cystic lesions is not uncommon in the early weeks of therapy. Improvement continues for several months after the period of treatment is completed. Occasionally a second course of treatment is necessary for maximum improvement. One of the obvious actions of isotretinoin is to decrease markedly the oil-gland size and the production of sebum—hence, to produce extremely dry skin.

Acne Surgery

The removing of blackheads with a special instrument designed for that task, and the opening of pustules and cysts, fall under a therapeutic technique that is called acne surgery. Although there may be immediate cosmetic improvements from these procedures, the long-term benefits are disputable. As a consequence, there are many competent and sincere dermatologists who perform surgery at regular intervals on their acne patients, and also many equally devoted doctors who do not believe in surgical intervention at all for the condition. All agree, however, that under no circumstances should patients perform their own versions of acne surgery. The results can be catastrophic, with infection and permanent scarring a not-uncommon end result.

Summary of Treatments

Over the years, various new treatments for acne have been greeted with enthusiasm, only to be discarded when it became apparent that they were worthless. It requires only a modest historical perspective not to become carried away with the current expectations for such medications as vitamin E and zinc. Not many years ago, large doses of vitamin A were very much in vogue in acne therapy, but today oral vitamin A is rarely prescribed. Similarly, injections of vaccine made from the staphylococcus bacteria, a frequent cause of boils and other skin infections, were once widely used for no logical reason, since these bacteria have never been shown to play a part in the acne process.

Some doctors continue to prescribe treatments of doubtful value. This is not dishonesty. It simply illustrates how difficult it is to determine the therapeutic value of a medicine used for a condition that has its ups and downs with or without medical attention.

Dermatologists have strong opinions about the medications they believe are effective against acne in its various stages. Some basic guidelines for treatment are outlined below. There is room for disagreement, and the overlap of treatments is obvious.

Mild Acne: External medications only. Over-the-counter products containing sulfur, salicylic acid, and benzoyl peroxide; medicated soaps; and the prescription topicals such as tretinoin, antibiotic lotions, and gels.

Moderate Acne: Above, plus oral antibiotics.

Severe Acne: Above, plus corticosteroids (orally and injected into acne cysts) and isotretinoin.

Acne Scars: Dermabrasion

Today acne therapy has improved to the extent that it can limit the severity of scarring in severe cystic acne. Nevertheless, after the acne process has burned itself out, many young people are left with permanent scars, ranging from a few insignificant depressions to multiple large scars and deep "ice pick" holes.

Dermabrasion, or facial planing, is a restorative, operative procedure that has been widely used to reduce the extent of acne scarring. It is an operation that is usually performed months or even years after the acne has become inactive, either in a doctor's office or in a hospital.

The initial step in dermabrasion is to freeze the skin with a chemical refrigerant. Once the skin is frozen hard, the superficial layers are removed by the light application of a rapidly spinning wire brush or diamond burr. The dermabraded skin after treatment appears red and moist as if the skin had suffered a second-degree burn.

Successful dermabrasion removes the epidermis and some of the dermis, but a portion of the hair follicles and oil glands is left behind to provide a source of cells that can regenerate to form a new smooth surface. In most cases, it is not possible to abrade to the full depth of all the scars, since this would remove all the tissue that usually provides cells for normal skin healing. This is the most obvious limitation of the dermabrasion procedure.

The postoperative treatment is variable, depending upon the philosophy of the operator. Healing takes a number of weeks in any case, and the skin remains red and extremely sensitive to sun and wind for many months. Often more than one dermabrasion is necessary to obtain maximum improvement.

At one time there was a great deal of enthusiasm for dermabrasion. This has been tempered over the years by the results, which are not that impressive, as well as an increased awareness of possible complications. These side effects may include alterations in skin pigmentation, yellow bumps on the skin due to oil-duct blockage, and, what is most disturbing, the appearance of keloids, which are areas of thickened, overdeveloped scar tissue.

Furthermore, dermabrasion, like many other cosmetic surgical procedures, often appeals to individuals whose problems are more than skin deep. Some teenagers and young adults persist in imagining that the elimination of their acne scars through dermabrasion will solve unrelated personal difficulties. Experienced dermatologists who regularly perform this procedure often attempt to dissuade these individuals from undergoing a treatment that may leave them disappointed and frustrated in the long run.

Thus, a few words of advice are in order for the reader who is contemplating dermabrasion. First of all: Wait! Time and patience go a long way in solving the problem of acne scarring. Mother Nature does a very creditable job in eliminating, or at least reducing, scars through natural healing and remodeling of the bumps and depressions. It is strongly recommended that patients wait at least one year from the time that acne lesions have stopped appearing so as to allow natural healing to take place before they contemplate dermabrasion.

Even after a suitable period of time has elapsed, do not make a decision to undergo this procedure without first obtaining an impartial, professional opinion from a knowledgeable dermatologist or plastic surgeon, preferably someone other than the one who will perform the procedure.

If the consulting doctor believes that dermabrasion is indicated, you should become thoroughly familiar with all the details of the procedure before making a final decision. You should know all the possible complications, and should also understand the maximum degree of improvement that can reasonably be expected.

Future Acne Treatments

If available treatment does not cure acne, and present surgical techniques are not always successful in eliminating acne scars, is there any hope in the future for acne sufferers? The answer is clearly yes. New forms of treatment are continually being developed, and isotretinoin is a case in point. Currently, research into the use of anti-androgens looks promising. Anti-androgens are chemicals that block the stimulating effect of androgens on the oil glands. Of course, anti-androgens cannot be administered systemically because of their possible harmful effects on other organs, but there is some hope that locally applied preparations might be effective in reducing acne.

With an increased understanding of the behavior of the skin and particularly of the sebaceous glands, it seems inevitable that there will soon be a new and more satisfactory way of handling the acne dilemma. Even today, available treatment can control acne to the point where permanent scarring can be largely prevented.

5 SKIN ALLERGIES

Allergies make for good cocktail party conversation. They are commonplace (if you don't have one, your friend does), they are often unpleasant but rarely life-threatening, and there is something mildly amusing about allergic symptoms, particularly if they are not *your* symptoms.

Most people have a distorted idea about the nature of allergies. There is an almost universal misconception, for instance, that allergic reactions can occur the first time a medication is swallowed, injected, or inhaled. An inaccurate corollary has it that a medication taken once or twice without allergic complications is forever safe. This is not the case. A reaction to any foreign substance—medication, food, or cosmetics—never occurs on the first exposure. It may take repeated encounters over a period of months, or even years, for the immune system to perceive that the substance is foreign and should be eliminated from the body. Only then will it mobilize the reaction that produces allergic symptoms. Keep it in mind: *Anybody* can become allergic to *any* foreign material at *any* time.

Another familiar misstatement: "My father is allergic to penicillin, so I guess I am also." Again, this is not true. The tendency to allergic reactions may be inherited, but *specific* allergies are not. It is also true that allergies are very reproducible—if you develop hives and blame it on shrimp cocktail, the next time you have shrimp cocktail you should experience hives; if you don't, then the first attack of hives was caused by something other than shrimp. Finally, allergic reactions are not dose related; a little bit can be as bad as a lot. One unit or one milligram of penicillin can cause as serious a reaction in a susceptible person as a whole syringe full of the antibiotic.

In actuality, human beings have a double-barreled system of allergic response. An immediate reaction occurs when antibodies, which are protein substances that circulate in the blood, react with the antigen, a foreign material that has entered the body. Within a matter of minutes, particular symptoms become evident. For example, following a bee sting the bee venom rapidly reacts with the antibodies already present in the bloodstream, and itching and swelling occur at the sting site. In more severe reactions, hives rapidly appear over the entire body.

In contrast, the delayed type of allergic reaction takes two to three days to evolve after exposure to the allergy-producing antigen. In delayed allergies, the lymphocytes (white blood cells) rather than the antibodies are attracted to the area where the antigen has entered the body. The skin test used for the diagnosis of tuberculosis is a classic example of a delayed allergy. In a positive skin test, an extract of the tuberculosis bacteria injected into the skin attracts lymphocytes that release chemicals at the injection area. The reaction becomes apparent in forty-eight hours as a small red bump, indicating an allergy to the tuberculosis germ.

The skin is not the only organ of the body to experience the effects of allergic reactions, but it does display many forms of allergies in a particularly vivid fashion. Some of the most common allergic skin disorders are contact dermatitis, urticaria (hives), allergic rashes from medications, and allergic reactions to sunlight.

ALLERGIC CONTACT DERMATITIS

One of the most common ailments seen in a dermatologist's office are rashes that occur as an allergic reaction to substances coming into contact with the skin. In contrast to an allergic rash from a food or ingested medication (generally a symmetrical rash all over the body), the rash of allergic contact dermatitis appears *only where the offending substance touched the skin*. For example, allergy to a particular bath soap might cause a rash all over your body, but allergy to lipstick dye will cause a rash that is limited to your lips and perhaps the adjacent skin.

Poison Ivy

The rash that develops after touching the poison ivy plant is an example of allergic contact dermatitis and is the most common form of this disease in the United States. The poison ivy plant, *Rhus radicans,* contains a chemical that is a potent cause of allergic reactions in many people. The poison ivy rash usually appears forty-eight hours after contact with any part of the plant, and occasionally even after exposure to inert carriers of the plant's sap, such as clothing, shoes, or a household pet. Exposure to the smoke from burning poison ivy leaves also has been known to cause severe rashes in highly sensitive individuals.

Poison ivy produces a distinctive pattern of bumps and blisters. Exposure usually occurs when a person inadvertently brushes against the leaves, which deposit the plant's sap in a line or streak on the skin. Thus a linear, blistering, red rash on exposed parts of the body is suggestive of a plant allergy. In the United States, the plant in question can be poison ivy or the botanically and chemically related poison sumac or poison oak plants.

There are several misconceptions about poison ivy allergy that are equally inaccurate when applied to other forms of contact allergy. One popular misconception is that the allergic dermatitis will appear on *first* contact with the plant. This is not the case. At least one or more exposures are required before an individual becomes "sensitized." However, poison ivy happens to be such a potent allergy producer that many people will become allergic after the first contact with the plant, and the *next* exposure will cause the typical poison ivy rash. Even a conventional skin test, where minute amounts of plant oil are applied to the skin, will induce a state of allergy in one out of every ten people tested.

A second misconception concerns the apparent spread of

poison ivy from one area of the body to another. Despite the presence of large, fluid-filled blisters, poison ivy is *not* a contagious disease. The blister fluid, which is derived from the serum of blood, does not contain plant oil and cannot spread the dermatitis or "infect" another person. Poison ivy appears to be spreading because the rash takes several days to evolve, and depends upon the amount of plant oil deposited and the degree of sensitivity of the skin. With large amounts of plant oil, the rash may appear in twenty-four to forty-eight hours. Smaller traces of oil may not evoke a reaction for four to five days. Swelling and redness around the eyes is often the first sign of poison ivy because the skin in this area is thin and vulnerable. The appearance of the rash in new areas may actually indicate a second or third exposure from inert carriers of the plant extract or from oil that has been trapped under the fingernails.

A hot shower with strong soap after a day in the woods is not likely to prevent a case of poison ivy. Once contact has been made, the plant's sap reacts with the skin in a matter of minutes. The reaction is irreversible, and after twenty minutes the oil is fixed to the skin and cannot be removed by any means. It is true that soap and water can inactivate the chemical responsible for the rash, but invariably the preventive shower takes place too late.

A final mistaken idea held by many people concerns the value of "injections" for poison ivy. Most dermatologists believe that desensitization with injections (or with pills) containing small amounts of an extract of the plant does not provide protection from further attacks of the dermatitis. The only useful prophylaxis is a little botanical education. Anybody who experiences frequent and severe bouts of poison ivy should become familiar with the appearance of the *Rhus* plant (see Figure 4) and follow the familiar adage, "Leaves of three, leave them be."

Treatment

Cold compresses and calamine lotion are adequate local measures for mild poison ivy. The many over-the-counter lotions have no special properties that make them valuable in treat-

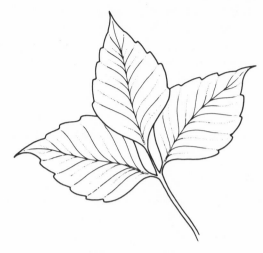

Figure 4. Poison ivy

ment. Although some of these preparations contain a chemical designed to relieve itching, they also can irritate the skin or even initiate another allergy on top of the original poison ivy. True, the widely prescribed corticosteroid lotions and creams provide more relief from itching than calamine lotion, but these expensive medications do not alter the normal course of the dermatitis, which lasts a distressingly long two to three weeks.

In very severe cases of poison ivy, it is possible to suppress the dermatitis with corticosteroid pills or injections. Corticosteroids decrease the allergic reaction and provide a less well-defined anti-inflammatory effect.

When given orally, corticosteroids are usually prescribed in a tapered dose schedule. Starting with a relatively large number of pills, the dose is decreased every one to two days over a two-week period. Although the rash clears completely within a few days, you must continue the treatment through the natural course of the disease. If you discontinue the treatment prematurely, the rash will recur. The tapered oral-corticosteroid schedule can be used in any severe form of allergic contact dermatitis, regardless of the specific allergen responsible.

There are many patients as well as many physicians who

believe that poison ivy dermatitis is a trivial problem and should not be treated with cortisone, a potent and potentially dangerous drug. But the fact remains that a severe case of poison ivy can be far more incapacitating than many more serious illnesses. It is certainly not a life-threatening disease, but, happily, the same can be said of most medical problems. Furthermore, a two-week regimen of corticosteroids is safe and almost free of complications, provided you are otherwise healthy.

Metal Allergy

Nickel, chromium, and mercury are the three metals that most frequently cause allergic contact dermatitis, nickel being the most common of the three. Allergy to gold, silver, and platinum is extremely rare. Allergic reactions to nickel can be a particularly annoying problem for women, since the metal is present in some jewelry, zippers, and clasps, as well as in many appliances and household utensils. During a day of normal activity, repeated contact with this metal is virtually unavoidable, although prolonged contact is more apt to produce an eruption. The presence of a rash on the earlobes, neck, or wrists suggests contact with nickel-containing jewelry, while a localized, itchy spot on the midback suggests a reaction to a nickel-containing brassiere fastener. One puzzling case of a symmetrical rash on the outside of the lower legs of one young woman turned out to be an allergy to the nickel zippers in her fashionable new boots.

Reactions to nickel can follow a seasonal pattern. Like most forms of contact dermatitis, intimacy of contact and the presence of moisture facilitate the development of the rash. There may be no signs of dermatitis in cold weather, but in a warm, humid environment, when the skin is persistently moist from perspiration, a rash can appear on the body at the sites of nickel contact.

As in the case of a poison ivy allergy, it is not possible to undo a nickel allergy with desensitization injections. When dressing up for a night on the town, however, a coat of clear nail polish or a corticosteroid cream applied to nickel-containing costume jewelry will provide you with protection for several hours.

Rubber Allergy

Allergy to rubber can lead to itching, redness, and blistering in some unexpected parts of the body. For instance, a rubber-sensitive student who chews on the eraser of his pencil may develop itchy lips, while a corpulent woman may have an extensive rash on her body from her elastic foundation garments. The feet are perhaps the most common location for rubber rash, not only from rubber-soled shoes, but more often from the rubber cement that welds the shoe parts together. Occasional cases of dermatitis in the genital area have been traced to an allergy to rubber contraceptive devices.

Rubber, like nickel, is a material so widely used in our society that it is difficult to avoid. But if the rubber-sensitive person is to remain free of rash, avoidance is the treatment of choice.

Hair Dye Allergy

Black dyes, based on the chemical paraphenylenediamine, are often used to color hair and furs. Hair dye allergies cause swelling and blistering of the scalp, the back of the neck, and the face. Like poison ivy, such allergic reactions can be so severe that treatment with a systemic corticosteroid is not only justified but necessary. Black dye allergy can cause a phenomenon called *cross-sensitization* that can have far-reaching consequences for the sufferer. Cross-sensitization means that if an allergy develops to substance A, and substance B has a similar chemical structure, then an allergic rash will probably occur on exposure to either A or B. This cross-sensitivity makes it possible for a person to have multiple allergies from sensitization to only one compound.

In the case of the dye paraphenylenediamine, cross-sensitization may occur not only with other similar dyes, but with several chemically similar medications, including anesthetics that have "-caine" in their names; the sulfa drugs; and a chemical called para-aminobenzoic acid (PABA), which is used extensively in sunscreen preparations. A case in point: A patient recovering from a severe scalp rash due to black dye allergy went on a vacation to forget her problem, only to develop a similar rash on her face when she applied her favorite sunscreen lotion containing PABA. The only conclusion is an allergy to paraphenylenediamine with cross-sensitization to PABA.

Cosmetic Allergy

The paraphenylenediamine hair-dye reaction is an example of a cosmetic allergy. The overall incidence of allergic reactions to other cosmetic preparations is surprisingly low considering the great variety and widespread use of cosmetics, perfume, body lotions, and hair products. The most obvious reason for this is that the cosmetic industry screens all new products for allergy-producing properties. However, the number of tested volunteers is limited, and the real test ultimately takes place in the open market, when the product is used by thousands of consumers.

Cosmetic reactions can evoke the single most common misconception about allergies. "It can't be due to the eye makeup," says the woman with the red, swollen eyes. "I've been using the same product for the last ten years." Unfortunately, this is not true. The human immune system sometimes operates in strange and mysterious ways. Even after ten years of regular use, the immune system may decide that the eye makeup is objectionable, and the swollen eyes become the allergy system's message of rejection. The fact that months or even years may elapse before the reaction appears is an accepted but unexplained phenomenon.

Of course, there is another reason for a delayed reaction to a cosmetic. Although the names of products remain constant, their ingredients may change. For this reason, yesterday's routinely used eyeliner may become tomorrow's allergen. How often does the consumer take the time to read the list of ingredients in a cosmetic preparation? For that matter, government regulations notwithstanding, how often are all the contents listed?

A rigid approach to the detection of a specific cause of cosmetic dermatitis is often not welcomed by the patient. Most women would like their physician to single out only one cosmetic as the most likely cause of their problem. Since a diagnosis then becomes a matter of educated guesswork, the doctor would prefer that all cosmetics be discontinued until the rash clears. Once the dermatitis has disappeared, one can resume using the cosmetics one at a time, adding a new preparation every three to four days. If signs of a recurrent rash appear, the most recently added cosmetic is the likely cause of the allergy. This form of "use testing" is often a more practical approach than the more elaborate, time-consuming patch testing that is discussed below. Since some cosmetics contain multiple ingredients, however, it may be necessary to rely on patch testing to determine the *specific* ingredient that caused the allergy, and to prevent recurrent rashes from other cosmetics with the same ingredient.

The "hypoallergenic" (less allergy-producing) cosmetics are occasionally helpful to patients with cosmetic sensitivity. These products are very similar to the standard brands but lack the perfume and other chemicals that frequently cause allergic reactions. There are no specially prepared cosmetics that eliminate all sources of allergy, however, and for many, the avoidance of all cosmetics may be the only practical solution to severe and continuing cosmetic dermatitis. Thus, the "natural" look often becomes a necessary part of the treatment.

Finding the Cause

Dermatologists often are able to figure out the specific cause of allergic contact dermatitis based upon their knowledge and experience with common sensitizing chemicals likely to come into contact with particular areas of the body. Although one rash may look like another, a distinctive distribution of the disorder on the body can provide clues to the diagnosis. A rash on the earlobes is likely to be caused by an allergy to the nickel present in earrings, to a perfume applied behind the ears, or to a hair preparation, while an eyelid dermatitis suggests an allergy to eye makeup, medicated eye drops, or even nail polish. (Touching the skin around the eyes with lacquered fingernails is sufficient to provoke dermatitis in this sensitive area in some people.) The table below is a partial list of some of the common patterns of allergic contact dermatitis.

COMMON CONTACT ALLERGENS

If you have a rash on:	*You may be allergic to:*
Face	Soaps, cosmetics, hair dye, hair spray, lanolin, shampoo, depilatories, aerosol sprays, pollen
Mouth	Dental cleansers, mouthwash, lipstick, chewing gum, food dyes
Ears	Jewelry (nickel), perfume, glasses, hair dye
Eyes	Nail polish, cosmetics, eye drops, eyelash curlers
Hands	Paper, dyes, natural foods, food additives, soap, perfume, nickel, rubber, occupational contact agents
Feet	Nickel, chromium, leather, dyes, rubber
Body	Synthetic fabrics, wash-and-wear clothing, dry-cleaning chemicals, soaps, detergents, dyes, rubber, elastic, cosmetics, powder
Any part of the body	Medications applied to the skin

If the cause of the allergic reaction cannot be determined by your medical history or the distribution of the rash on your body, patch testing offers another diagnostic method that may solve the puzzle. A patch test is essentially an attempt to reproduce the contact dermatitis on a small scale. Materials selected for testing are applied to your skin (usually on the back) and covered with a dressing or patch. After forty-eight to seventy-two hours—the usual incubation period for contact dermatitis—the patches are removed and the test sites are examined for signs of an allergic reaction: redness, swelling of the skin, blistering, or a combination of all three.

The patch test method is scientifically sound, but it is not foolproof, and several pitfalls must be kept in mind. One is that although there are many test materials available that encompass most common allergies, the unknown offending material may not be considered a likely cause of the rash, and therefore will not be included in the tests. If this is the case, the test is useless. Furthermore, patch testing frequently turns up "incidental" positive tests that can be misleading. Patients who suffer from contact dermatitis often have more than one allergy, and one or more positive tests may be entirely unrelated to the problem at hand.

Finally, there are those rare occasions when your skin will not react to a material in the manner in which it is applied in the patch-testing procedure, but the same substance will still give you a rash if exposure occurs in a more natural manner. Still, this aberration is rare if the patch tests are prepared and applied correctly.

As long as the physician and the patient are aware of these shortcomings, patch testing is a valuable diagnostic tool when other techniques have failed to turn up the cause of the allergic rash. The most effective treatment of allergic contact dermatitis consists of avoidance of the offending substance (the allergen) and general care of the inflamed skin (see chapter 2).

Allergies to Medications

Topical Medications Allergic rashes frequently arise from self-treatment with some popular over-the-counter topical medications. The following scenario describes a series of events that happens all too frequently.

The patient-to-be (hereafter known as "P") develops a minor but uncomfortable skin irritation. P consults his friendly neighborhood pharmacist, who recommends the use of an anti-itch lotion containing an antihistamine or perhaps one of the anesthetic "-caine" drugs: benzocaine, tetracaine, or butycaine. Unfortunately, these medications can cause allergic rashes, particularly if they are repeatedly rubbed into skin that is already red and inflamed.

At first P experiences some relief from the itching, but after a few days he notices that what started as a minor skin irritation has become more severe. P steps up his treatment with the anti-itch lotion, and as he does so, the rash spreads and becomes worse. This is interpreted by P as a signal to escalate his therapeutic activity even further.

Sooner or later P must seek medical attention. The dermatologist, who is very familiar with this self-help syndrome, will recognize that the original itch has been completely obscured by a severe allergic rash from an ingredient in the anti-itch lotion, and will quickly interrupt the patient's self-destructive cycle.

It is important for all self-medicators to be aware that their problems can be caused by many topical medications that are readily available with or without a prescription. A partial list would include: iodine, mercury-containing antiseptics, antibiotics such as penicillin or neomycin, and sulfonamides, as well as antihistamines and "-caine" anesthetics. These medications are less likely to cause allergic reactions if taken in pill form or by injection.

Internal Medications Allergic reactions from drugs taken orally are so varied that it is impossible to describe all the multiplicity of colors, shapes, and sites of possible skin rashes that can develop. These drug reactions are notable not only because of their variety but because they mimic many common skin disorders such as psoriasis, eczema, and even acne. Unfortunately, as the number of medications that are prescribed increases, the problem of drug allergy expands proportionately. A corollary to the allergy rule applies here: Any medication can cause almost any allergic rash at any time. There are few exceptions to this general statement. Some medications, such as milk of magnesia and digitalis, are considered to be safe drugs and never cause an allergic reaction, but few drugs fall into this category.

Finding the Cause Determining the cause of a drug reaction in patients who are taking several medications can become a complex diagnostic problem. Since there are no routine skin or blood tests that can pinpoint the specific drug causing the allergy, diagnosis becomes a matter of evaluating the statistical odds. Physicians must become familiar with the allergic potential of hundreds of medications and the varied spectrum of their reactions. Sometimes the problem is a simple one and the odds overwhelmingly point to one medication. If you develop hives while taking penicillin, an antihistamine, vitamins, and milk of magnesia, it is more than likely that the penicillin is the cause of your problem. Penicillin can often cause allergic reactions, particularly hives, while the other medications rarely cause allergies of any kind.

Statistical diagnosis is aided by the fact that the skin shows some common patterns of reaction that are associated with a particular group of medications. These drugs are the most frequent causes of the rash. For example, urticaria (hives) is often an allergic reaction to penicillin, sulfa drugs, or barbiturates, while blistering rashes are due to bromides or iodine-containing medications and to some of the medicines that are used to treat epilepsy. Purpura (bleeding into the skin) can be caused by sulfa drugs, quinine or quinidine, and gold, while eczema-like reactions occur with penicillin, streptomycin, and some of the tranquilizers. Lists of this nature, however, are of only limited value in making a statistical diagnosis because drugs are unpredictable in their effects on people.

The "fixed" drug reaction is one of the more unusual forms of allergic response to a medication. The rash appears (is fixed) to one or two limited areas of the skin. The afflicted areas become swollen and turn a striking reddish-purple color within hours after the medication is ingested. The remarkable feature of the fixed drug reaction is that the same areas of the skin react with the same rash when the causative drug is administered days or even months after the original reaction. The following case history illustrates this most unusual form of allergy:

A man consulted a dermatologist because he experienced a purplish swelling on the right side of his forehead following his regular visit to a psychiatrist. Both the patient and the psychiatrist were of the opinion that the skin eruption was an "emotional reaction," a sign of anxiety caused by the psychotherapeutic sessions. Although the patient vehemently denied taking any medication, the dermatologist suggested that the swellings might represent a fixed drug reaction. When this possibility was brought to the attention of the psychiatrist, it became apparent that the skin rash occurred only after those sessions in which the psychiatrist gave the patient an injection of amobarbital, a barbiturate drug. As soon as the injections were discontinued, the so-called emotional swellings ceased.

In addition to barbiturates, some common causes of fixed drug reactions include the antibiotic tetracycline; a chemical called phenolphthalein, found in some laxatives; and the painkiller phenacetin.

At times it is the patient who unwittingly hinders a diagnosis of a drug reaction. Some patients simply forget they are taking medications while others do not consider certain drugs to be "true" medicines. To some women, birth control medication is simply "the pill," not a medication. Aspirin, vitamin pills, eye and nose drops, tonics, and laxatives are similarly dismissed. Yet all of these substances can cause allergic reactions. In the context of drug allergy, any material other than food taken through any of the body orifices should be considered a medication.

Treatment for Allergic Drug Reactions The first step in the treatment of all allergic drug reactions is the obvious one: discontinue the causative medication. There are times when this is not as simple as it sounds; the offending medication may be lifesaving or at least important in maintaining a person's health. However, often there are medications available that are chemically different from the offending drug that can serve as satisfactory substitutes. Or, occasionally, a drug reaction can be tolerated and the medication continued, although this can have dangerous consequences if the allergic reaction affects the kidneys or some other vital organs.

In situations where multiple medications are involved, one can play the odds and discontinue the drugs that are most likely to cause the allergic reactions. In the case of very severe allergic reactions, however, it may be necessary to immediately discontinue all medications.

Treatment of a drug allergy rash with symptom-reducing medication will provide some comfort, but it does not shorten the duration of the reaction, which continues until all of the offending drug has been inactivated or excreted from the body. Antihistamines are most useful in the treatment of hivelike drug reactions, and they provide some relief from the itching associated with many other forms of allergic drug reactions. The unpleasant symptoms associated with drug rashes can be suppressed with large doses of corticosteroids until the reaction has run its course. This treatment, however, is usually reserved for those suffering from the most severe forms of allergy, and only for those patients who are unlikely to suffer serious side effects from this potent group of drugs.

Allergy to the Sun

Fair-skinned people believe they are "allergic" to the sun because they tend to experience severe burns after minor sun exposure. But this form of hypersensitivity is related to a relative lack of protective melanin pigment, and not to the actions of antibodies and lymphocytes, as in the case of true allergy.

Both fair- and dark-skinned people, however, can become allergic to the sun and can develop hives or other forms of itchy rashes on exposed portions of the skin immediately following exposure to sunlight. Most of these sun-induced reactions are short-lived and clear up soon after the sun exposure is eliminated.

The first line of defense against sun allergy is prevention. The sun-allergic person may choose to avoid sun exposure altogether, or else use a protective sunscreening lotion or cream when outdoors. For reactions to short-wave ultraviolet light, use sunscreens containing PABA. If the sensitizing rays are long-wave ultraviolet, protective lotions containing benzophenones are worth a try. A better choice might be one of the completely opaque sunscreens that block out all visible and ultraviolet light by their reflective properties (see chapter 11). Regardless of the choice, sunscreens rarely provide complete protection and you should reserve them for minimal, unavoidable sun exposure rather than for prolonged sunbathing, a practice that should be avoided.

Sometimes sunlight, in conjunction with a medication, can induce an allergic reaction in an individual. If the medication is taken without exposure to the sun, then no rash appears—sun exposure without the medication similarly will not produce a rash. It is the combination of medication and sunshine that can create the allergy that tends to show up as a rash on the face, the open-collar portion of the chest, the tops of the arms, and, in fact, in all areas of the skin exposed directly to sunlight. These photo-allergic drug reactions can occur in patients who take some frequently prescribed, chemically similar drugs, the sulfonamide antibiotics and the diuretic hydrochlorothiazide, as well as some of the oral medications used to treat diabetes. The tetracycline antibiotics and a family of tranquilizers, the phenothiazines, are also known for their ability to cause sun reactions.

Some chemicals cause sun sensitivity when they come into contact with sun-exposed areas of the body. These external photosensitizers are found naturally in fruits such as the lime, in many plants of the carrot family, and artificially in some perfumes and cosmetics. As in the case of medications, sunlight alone or the chemical alone, without sun exposure, will not trigger the allergic reaction; it is the combination of the two that causes rashes in the sun-exposed areas.

The most frequent form of sun sensitivity results in a diverse group of rashes that are called the *polymorphous light eruptions*. The word *polymorphous* means "many forms" and indeed these reactions may appear on the skin as blisters, flat spots, or small hives. Although the cause of these rashes is not known, they are not due to true allergy in the technical sense, since antibodies play no role in their origin.

Polymorphous light eruptions appear on the sun-exposed skin after the first sun exposure of the spring or early summer. If the sun exposure continues, so does the rash. If sunlight is eliminated, the rash gradually fades away. Occasionally there is a lessening in the severity of the rash, or even a complete clearing as the summer wears on, despite continued exposure to the sun.

Treatment The cause of this form of sun sensitivity is unknown and treatment at best only relieves the symptoms. For diehard sun worshippers, the sunscreen preparations on the market may modify but rarely eliminate the rash. There are a group of internal medications used to treat malaria that are useful in preventing polymorphous light eruptions—if they are taken on a regular basis. These are potent medications, however, with sometimes serious side effects. They should be reserved for those situations where sun exposure cannot be avoided, and not for casual sunbathing.

Urticaria (Hives)

A hive is an itchy, red, or skin-colored swelling that usually comes and goes in a matter of hours. (A swelling that persists for several days is not likely to be a hive.) A solitary hive of this type can be an allergic response to an insect bite, a plant, or any other foreign substance that scratches or penetrates the skin. Multiple hives, collectively called *urticaria,* are usually caused by an internal allergic reaction and can last for a number of days, even weeks.

This type of urticaria is frequently due to an allergy to a food or medication. Chocolate, nuts, fish, eggs, and pork are several of the most common foods that cause allergies, while penicillin is one of the leading medicines that is apt to produce hives in certain individuals. There are still other foods and medications, including shellfish, strawberries, and aspirin, that may cause hives, not because of allergic reactions, but because they contain chemicals that stimulate the body to activate histamine. (Histamine is the chemical that alters the integrity of the blood vessels in such a way that serum leaks out and puddles under the skin, forming the hive swelling.)

Dermatologists and allergists have discovered that occasionally some "hivers" may be reacting to chemical additives such as preservatives, dyes, and artificial flavorings often found in food, medications, and even toothpastes. The principal offenders are the salicylates and benzoates, which are chemically similar to ordinary aspirin. These problem additives are found in a wide variety of edibles including candy, puddings and pie fillings, pickles and condiments, cakes and other baked goods, bologna, and wine. Hive-producing synthetic dyes and artificial colors are widely used in soft drinks, frozen desserts, cake icing, and even the coating of pills and capsules that are used to treat hives. A ten-day trial of a natural food diet consisting of unadulterated cereal, flour, eggs, meat, chicken, rice, and potatoes is one way of determining if chemical additives are responsible for persistent and otherwise unexplained hives.

Most physicians are reluctant to do extensive skin testing to search for the elusive cause of hives, largely because the results are often misleading, with many "positive" tests that clearly have no relationship to the hives. A painless and less expensive method to resolve the question of food allergy is a *diet diary*. You are instructed to keep a careful record of all foods and medications ingested, and to record the times the hives appear. After two weeks, your doctor analyzes the diary and tries to correlate the appearance of the hives with the ingestion of specific foods. For example, urticaria developed in an obese woman shortly after she started a high-protein, weight-reduction diet. The hives appeared regularly an hour or two after most meals. Analysis of a relatively simple diet diary suggested that tuna fish was the cause of the problem, since it appeared on the menu at lease once or twice daily. It was recommended that tuna be dropped from the diet, but the hives continued to appear. At this point it became obvious that the only food common to almost all meals was a diet soft drink, but flavors and brands varied. All diet drinks and artificial sweeteners were then eliminated from the diet, and the hives disappeared. When the patient inadvertently drank a diet cola drink, the hives recurred, again confirming the specific cause of the eruption.

The *elimination diet* is another method for investigating food allergies. In one method, foods that are suspect can be eliminated a few at a time—a tedious, time-consuming process. A better approach is to place the patient on a radically restricted diet. For example, you would be instructed to eat four low-allergy foods—lamb, rice, apples, and tea. No other food is permitted for a period of seven days. (You must be truly desperate to tolerate this repetitious diet, but at least it serves to put the food allergy question to rest.) If the hives continue in their regular pattern, then it is safe to conclude that food has nothing to do with your urticaria. If the hives disappear (a rare event), then new foods can be introduced into your diet one at a time in order to pinpoint the specific food or foods that are the hive makers. If your condition becomes much worse (an even rarer event), then one of the low-allergy diet foods must be considered as a probable cause of your persistent urticaria.

Skin testing, diet diaries, and elimination diets are reserved for the minority of patients who have hives that last for months or even years. Allergy to food or medication is rarely the cause of chronic hives. When an explanation for persistent urticaria is discovered, it may turn out that some internal disease such as arthritis, or an unsuspected infection such as that caused by intestinal parasites, has triggered the hives. Consequently, many chronic "hivers" are subjected to a battery of expensive laboratory tests in the hope of finding the obscure disease that will explain away the hives. Unfortunately, the cause of persistent hives can be found in less than 50 percent of patients.

Cold, heat, and even pressure can cause hives in some people with "physical" allergies. In a condition called *dermographism,* stroking or writing on the skin with a blunt object will produce hivelike lines within a few minutes. This form of pressure urticaria is usually a passing inconvenience, but occasionally there are dermographic individuals who find that they are unable to grasp a steering wheel or a tennis racquet without developing incapacitating itching and swelling of the hands.

Hives from allergies to cold also tend to be a short-lived problem unless they are associated with a blood disease or are of a rare hereditary form. Cold-induced hives can occur even with modest changes in environmental temperature. The transition, for instance, from a hot shower to a room-temperature bathroom, or a plunge into a tepid swimming pool on a hot day, can sometimes activate "cold" hives. Antihistamine medications are used to suppress this reaction, and "desensitization" through exposure to warm baths of gradually decreasing temperature is sometimes helpful.

Emotional disturbances are a favorite explanation for persistent hives when there is no other apparent cause. Although the role that anxiety plays in causing hives is greatly overemphasized, there are rare instances where emotional factors appear to trigger hive outbreaks. It also has been said that there is a distinctive time pattern for psychogenic urticaria. During the day, the skin remains relatively clear. Early in the evening hives begin to appear, and by bedtime they are in full bloom, ensuring a sleepless night. This cycle repeats itself day after day unless it is interrupted by treatment.

Treatment Although the cause of hives frequently is unexplained, the symptoms can be suppressed with an appropriate medication. The antihistamines are without question the most reliable drugs for this purpose. If one antihistamine proves ineffective, another of these chemically varied compounds will usually do the job if the prescribed dose is adequate.

There are several antihistamines to choose from, including the widely prescribed diphenhydramine, tripelennamine, chlorpheniramine, and hydroxyzine. Drowsiness is the major complaint that patients have when using these medications. (Terfenadine is a new antihistamine that doesn't cause drowsiness, but it is not quite as effective as the others.)

Some forms of hives are associated with swelling of the soft tissues underneath the skin and the lining of the mouth and throat—a condition called *angioneurotic edema.* If the internal swelling interferes with breathing or swallowing, it can turn into a medical emergency that requires immediate treatment with an injection of Adrenalin and sometimes corticosteroids. The corticosteroids are also helpful in eliminating persistent hives that do not respond to one of the antihistamine drugs.

Home treatment of hives with cool baths and lotions helps to relieve the itching but does little to change the pattern of eruption.

6 THE SKIN AND NUTRITION

Skin diseases resulting from poor nutrition are fortunately rare in our society. It is not difficult for most of us to fulfill our daily nutritional requirements—food supplies are abundant and even many processed foods are reinforced with vitamins, minerals, and other nutrients.

One current nutritional controversy concerns the value of vitamins and other supplements for healthy people who maintain a well-balanced diet. While the proponents of nutritional supplements believe they foster good health, others consider vitamins and minerals in excess of daily requirements as worthless and at times definitely detrimental to one's health.

The skin is a natural laboratory for this debate, since it is one of the first organs to reflect a deficiency or excess of vitamins in the body. Furthermore, nutritional cosmetologists are frequently in the news, often promoting their attempts to change the skin's appearance by altering the diet or by applying nutrients from the outside. Many people rely heavily on their advice—perhaps taking megadoses of vitamins and minerals regularly as part of their daily regime, or by using salves and creams reinforced with vitamins and other substances. This advice is frequently worthless and, in the case of vitamins and minerals, actually can be harmful.

VITAMINS

Vitamins are substances that the body uses in very small amounts to carry out many of its most critical metabolic reactions. For the most part, vitamins must be obtained from diet because your body is not capable of manufacturing them in adequate amounts in order to maintain health.

Vitamins are categorized into two groups: fat-soluble and water-soluble. The fat-soluble vitamins are A, D, E, and K; the water-soluble group includes the B-complex vitamins and vitamin C. One of the most important distinctions between the two groups is that the body can build up stores of only the fat-soluble vitamins for future use. Consequently, regular intake of foods containing water-soluble vitamin C and B-complex vitamins is a necessity, while intermittent intake of the fat-soluble group is well tolerated by your body. On the other hand, you can accumulate unhealthy amounts of fat-soluble vitamins in the body by consistently ingesting daily "supplements" that exceed the normal requirements. Let's take a look at the most commonly used vitamins and minerals and see how both deficient and excess quantities of each affect your skin.

Vitamin A

Vitamin A (retinol) is present in substantial amounts in liver and dairy products; it is also contained, in a precursor form (beta carotene), in yellow and green vegetables such as carrots and squash. Vitamin A is extremely important in maintaining healthy epithelial cells, such as the epidermis. In vitamin-A deficiency, the skin becomes overkeratinized, an abnormality called *phrynoderma*. In this condition, the skin appears dry and scaly, and small papules develop around the openings of the hair follicles, creating a rough graterlike texture.

Eye changes usually precede or accompany these skin abnormalities—night blindness may be an early symptom of vitamin-A deficiency. More serious eye changes, due to a drying of the superficial cells, develop if vitamin-A deficiency persists. If the condition is recognized early, both your skin and eye abnormalities can be reversed in a matter of months by administering vitamin A in doses *somewhat greater* than the daily requirement of 5,000 units.

Vitamin A is stored in the liver; thus, it is possible for you to build up large amounts of it in your body by taking regular doses that exceed the normal daily requirement. Some food faddists attempt to store up vitamin A by eating large quantities of carrots or squash. Fortunately, since these foods provide only beta carotene, the only ill effect of this excessive intake is a yellowish discoloration of the skin that can be seen vividly on their palms, the soles of their feet, and their faces. This condition is called *carotenemia,* a term describing an excessive amount of a yellow carotenoid pigment in the bloodstream. The color will fade once the excessive intake of beta carotene terminates.

More serious problems develop if you take synthetic vitamin A orally in doses that far exceed daily requirements. Paradoxically, some of the observable skin changes that result from your taking excessive amounts of vitamin A are similar to the changes seen in the deficiency state—namely, dry, scaly skin. But far more serious abnormalities can occur in your nervous system from excessive intake of vitamin A than from a deficiency of the vitamin. The following case history illustrates this point: A nine-year-old boy was taken to a dermatologist because his mother had noted that the boy's hair was falling out. The doctor confirmed the hair loss and noted that the skin was excessively dry and scaly, and that the boy appeared lethargic and unsteady on his feet. Upon careful questioning, the mother indicated that during a six-month period she had given the boy a 25,000-unit vitamin-A supplement as well as a daily multivitamin tablet containing 5,000 units. A blood analysis confirmed the fact that the child was suffering from hypervitaminosis A. Fortunately, all of the symptoms disappeared in a matter of months when the vitamin-A "treatment" was discontinued.

The retinoids, a new class of drugs that are similar to vitamin A, represent a major advance in dermatological therapy. The retinoids currently in use include tretinoin (Retin-A) and the oral medications isotretinoin (Accutane) and etretinate (see chapters 4 and 11). Newer and safer retinoids are being investigated at this time by many pharmaceutical companies, and probably will reach the marketplace in the near future.

Vitamin E

It has been said that vitamin E is "a vitamin in search of a deficiency." Vitamin-E deficiency is extremely rare and is generally due to diseases that block its absorption from the gastrointestinal tract. Symptoms of vitamin-E deficiency include a rare form of anemia in infants and equally rare nervous-system problems in adults.

Rats on diets deficient in vitamin E develop sterility. This observation has not been confirmed in humans, but the finding has encouraged some misguided individuals to take large doses of vitamin E to increase their sexual potency. To some extent the medical profession has supported the vitamin-E folly. Large doses of vitamin E have been recommended by some physicians and nutritionists for the treatment of a number of skin diseases, heart disease, muscular disorders, and even cancer, without the compelling evidence needed to support its beneficial effects in these conditions.

Patients often take it upon themselves to rub the contents of vitamin-E capsules or vitamin-E creams and lotions on skin rashes, acne, wounds, and scars. Except for the occasional allergic reaction, no harm has been reported from the topical use of vitamin E. In contrast, overdosing by the oral route can block the absorption of other fat-soluble vitamins, such as A and D.

The natural sources of vitamin E are vegetable oils, including wheat germ oil. The daily requirement is rather arbitrarily set at twelve to fifteen international units, an amount that is provided by natural foods in the average American diet.

Vitamin D

The skin is extremely important in helping to fulfill the vitamin-D requirements of the body. All of our daily needs of this vitamin can be manufactured in the skin through a chemical reaction that uses ultraviolet or natural sunlight as a source of energy. In the wintertime, when there is insufficient sun exposure, signs of vitamin-D deficiency can develop in some children who are not given adequate D supplements, although this is a rare condition.

Rickets, a serious bone disease, also can be prevented by adequate amounts of vitamin D in the diet. Rickets is almost nonexistent in the United States today because most cows' milk is reinforced with synthetic vitamin D in sufficient quantities to provide the daily 400 international units required for infants and growing children. Older children and adults require less vitamin D because the growth and calcification of their bones have been completed.

Vitamin K

The public appears to show very little interest in vitamin K, possibly because vitamin-K deficiency from inadequate dietary intake is virtually unheard of. Vitamin K is present in green vegetables, but most of the individual daily needs are provided by bacteria that manufacture K within the human intestine. Signs of deficiency develop in people who have liver or intestinal diseases that interfere with the normal passage of vitamin K from the inside of the intestine into the bloodstream.

Vitamin K is important in the normal formation of blood clots; therefore, the most obvious signs of deficiency are bleeding from the nose or rectum and hemorrhages under the skin. Many people with serious diseases of the heart or blood vessels are given medicines that are designed to interfere with blood clotting. If excessive bleeding occurs, the effects of some of these anticoagulant medications can be neutralized by injections of vitamin K.

B-Complex Vitamins

An inadequate intake of water-soluble vitamin B complex can result in a number of skin abnormalities. A deficiency of niacin, one of the B vitamins, is responsible for a disease called *pellagra,* a word derived from the Italian, meaning "rough skin." The pellagra rash often appears in the springtime, on areas of the skin exposed to sunshine. Diarrhea and mental disturbances are other prominent symptoms of this disease. In fact, medical students learn that there are four *D*s that characterize pellagra—dermatitis, diarrhea, dementia, and death. Pellagra is rare in the United States, although occasional cases are seen among chronic alcoholics. The disease occurs when alcohol provides all of a person's daily caloric requirements and the natural sources of niacin, such as meat and cereal grains, are not ingested.

Similarly, riboflavin (vitamin B_2) deficiency is unlikely to develop with a balanced diet containing meat, milk, and green vegetables. In fact, it takes prolonged starvation to induce the skin changes that are characteristic of riboflavin and other B-complex vitamin deficiencies. These symptoms include: redness, peeling, and cracking of the lips; dermatitis at the corners of the mouth; a sore, swollen tongue; and a scaly rash in the so-called seborrheic areas of the face. Seborrheic dermatitis itself is a very common skin disease that many thousands of Americans experience from time to time as ordinary dandruff of the scalp and a red scaly rash at the hairline, in the eyebrows, and adjacent to the nose (see chapter 2). But in otherwise healthy people, seborrheic dermatitis is not a reflection of riboflavin deficiency or any other form of vitamin deficiency. This fact has become evident over the years as many, many doses of B-complex vitamins have been administered to patients as treatment for seborrheic dermatitis, without success.

Vitamin B_{12} has also been overused and abused by some physicians for decades. Deficiency of this vitamin, caused by the body's inability to absorb it, results in pernicious anemia, which can be diagnosed by blood examinations. The only associated skin changes are extreme pallor—seen in most severe anemias—and a tender, swollen, smooth tongue. Because the early symptoms of pernicious anemia can be somewhat vague, some doctors have given B_{12} injections to treat fatigue, nervousness, and a number of ill-defined skin rashes. Many patients swear by their "B_{12} shots," but this treatment seems to be no more than placebo therapy. A diet that contains adequate amounts of protein is not likely to result in a B_{12} deficiency, providing the gastrointestinal tract is capable of absorbing the vitamin.

Vitamin C

Vitamin C (ascorbic acid) is the other water-soluble vitamin that is either immediately metabolized in the body or excreted. Regular intake of vitamin C is essential in maintaining the normal integrity of blood vessels. A prolonged deficiency of the vitamin leads to a disease called *scurvy*, in which bleeding into the skin and gums is the most striking symptom.

In the eighteenth century, scurvy was rampant among English soldiers and sailors who were forced to subsist on diets lacking in fresh fruits and vegetables. A Scottish naval surgeon recognized that scurvy could be prevented or cured by adding fresh citrus fruits to the sailors' diet.

In the past few years, large doses of vitamin C, sometimes in the thousands-of-milligrams range, have been recommended for the prevention or treatment of the common cold. But solid research studies are lacking to support such use of vitamin C in mild or acute respiratory diseases. Furthermore, since vitamin C is an acid, it is not altogether harmless—a caution that is important if you are prone to form kidney stones when your urine is acidified. Large doses of vitamin C can also cause diarrhea.

MINERALS

Little information is available about changes in the skin caused by diets deficient in the many minerals normally found in a balanced diet. Although an iron deficiency may cause nail abnormalities, most people who complain of brittle, lifeless nails do not have reduced levels of iron in their blood, and the nail ailment is usually due to some other undefined cause. Hair loss in women has also been attributed at times to iron deficiency, but correction of the problem with iron supplements does not ensure a regrowth of hair.

Zinc, a mineral required by the body in small quantities, has some dermatological significance. A rare intestinal and skin disease of infants, *acrodermatitis enteropathica*, can be cured by adding zinc to the diet. In the past few years, zinc has been recommended by some doctors for the treatment of acne as well. The effectiveness of zinc for this condition is difficult to evaluate, but it is certainly not the ultimate cure.

PROTEINS, FATS, AND CARBOHYDRATES

Your skin, like the other organs of your body, requires a diet that provides all the basic foods: proteins from meat, fish, fowl, dairy products, and legumes; fats from various oil sources and from many of the same foods that are rich in protein; and carbohydrates from sugar and starchy foods. Scientists today still know little about skin changes related to modest alterations in the amounts of proteins, fats, and carbohydrates consumed in the diet. Probably there are none. Certainly the basic human diet varies widely throughout the world, depending upon geographical and cultural differences, as well as the natural distribution and cultivation of foods. These wide variations in food consumption, however, cannot be linked to any consistent skin characteristics.

Alterations in the appearance of your skin do become apparent when you radically reduce the number of total calories you consume; the skin changes are due to an inadequate intake of proteins, fats, or carbohydrates, or all three. (Successful dieters, for instance, may notice that their skin often becomes dry, slack, and inelastic.) In cases of prolonged starvation, the skin would become rough, scaly, and subject to irritation or rashes. These changes could be accompanied by a mottled discoloration from areas of increased or decreased skin pigment. Profound protein starvation in very young children, a condition called *kwashiorkor,* can cause these skin changes as well as a distinctive reddish discoloration of the hair.

In the United States, the recent spate of popular rapid-weight-loss diets that are usually high in protein but low in fats and carbohydrates have not been associated with any obvious or consistent skin abnormalities. Many women who have been successful with these types of diets, however, have noticed a temporary but sometimes severe loss of hair, probably due to the fact that sudden weight loss deprives the rapidly dividing hair cells of protein, thus upsetting the normal hair cycle.

VITAMIN AND DIET THERAPY

Special diets for the treatment of skin disorders, especially those for which a specific cause has not been identified, have been tried for centuries. Diet therapy still has many advocates, but the results to date have not been impressive.

In the case of acne, patients formerly were handed a list of do-not-eats, whose selection depended largely on the prejudices of the doctor dispensing the list. Fried foods, chocolate, and other foods rich in fat were usually forbidden. It is now accepted that this restriction is a needless ban, since the sebaceous glands function independently of the amount of fat in the diet. We all know vegetarians with oily skin, and pizza eaters whose skin is dry and blemish-free.

Psoriasis is another chronic skin disease of unknown cause that frequently has been treated by diet manipulation. A low-fat diet and large doses of vitamin A or B complex have been recommended in the past without any scientific justification. In fact, several years ago adherents of these regimens claimed that psoriasis sufferers on an all-white-meat turkey diet experienced amazing "cures"—needless to say, turkey farmers became fat and prosperous. One day the scientific basis for this diet was challenged and the flimsy rationale behind it was totally disproven. It quickly became apparent that the dramatic "cures" were merely attributable to the ups and downs of this unpredictable disease.

Even dandruff, the most common manifestation of seborrheic dermatitis, has been subject to vitamin therapy by some physicians. Many doctors have been known to recommend vitamin-rich yeast cakes, vitamin-B-complex tablets, vitamin B_{12} injections, as well as instructing patients to drink six to ten glasses of water a day. No harm is done with this approach, but no obvious good, either.

FEEDING YOUR SKIN FROM THE OUTSIDE

Cosmeticians have long recommended to their clients the use of creams, salves, and ointments containing such delicacies as avocados, bananas, extracts of turtle, whale, mink, and wheat germ. The basic ingredient in all of these cosmetic aids is an oil of some sort. Without doubt this oil is what provides your skin with a smooth and supple feeling and acts as the effective moisture-retaining barrier. As for the other "nutrients" in these concoctions, it is highly unlikely that they can percolate down into your skin to the point where they can be utilized in its metabolic processes. It is also unproven and questionable whether vitamins or collagen put into various topical skin products are of any value when applied to the skin surface.

Tretinoin, a form of vitamin A, is an exception. Its effects on the superficial layers of the skin and the sebaceous gland ducts are of therapeutic value in the treatment of severe acne. Tretinoin has also recently been used for reversing some changes in the skin associated with sun damage, although not without some side effects (see chapter 11).

But, in general, the kindest appraisal of "skin food" would be simply to restate the nutritional verity that reflects both our ignorance and our wisdom: The proper feeding of your skin is accomplished by your ingesting a diet that is balanced in proteins, fats, and carbohydrates, and that contains the daily requirements of vitamins and essential minerals.

7 THE HAIR AND NAILS

HAIR

Several years ago, the author had the unique experience of participating in a hair-growing experiment. An amateur scientist had created a complex preparation that, when massaged into the scalp of balding men, was said to induce hair growth. Personal testimonials and photographs of balding men with newly growing hair were offered as evidence of the efficacy of this remarkable compound.

The mission was to design a study to confirm or refute the validity of the inventor's claim. A group of balding men were selected as candidates for the experiment. After careful hair counts and color photos of the scalp, the volunteers were subjected to a daily scalp massage with the new compound. After six months, new hair counts and further photographs determined that the hair-growing preparation did not grow hair.

The most interesting aspect of the hair-growing experiment was the misplaced optimism of many of the people involved in the project. From the very beginning, volunteers, scalp massagers, and other personnel were convinced that the material under investigation did initiate hair growth. The volunteers themselves offered frequent reports of their noticeable new hair growth that had been confirmed by friends and family.

At the end of the study, despite all evidence to the contrary, many of the participants were still convinced that they had grown hair. They went away miffed by the notion that a remarkable new product would never be marketed for public use. This type of wishful thinking is not at all unusual and, in fact, has supported for many years a multibillion-dollar industry that offers cosmetics, medications, and treatments for all sorts of hair problems.

For the consumer, an understanding of the normal behavior of hair is necessary in order to evaluate realistically the claims of the hair-treatment industry.

How Hair Grows

It is estimated that there are 100,000 hairs on the average human head, give or take a few thousand. In most animals, the function of hair appears to be one of protection and temperature regulation. In man, hair seems almost valueless except for its decorative properties.

Hair growth in animals and humans is a cyclic phenomenon. But the human hair cycle, unlike that of other mammals, is asynchronous, which means that each scalp hair is growing or has discontinued its growth phase independently of the activity of its neighboring hairs. This is cosmetically fortunate; otherwise, periodically, all your hair would fall out at the same time, as it does in some furry animals that undergo a seasonal molt.

The normal human hair cycle is divided into three phases: a period of growth called *anagen* (scalp hair grows at a rate of 0.3 to 0.4 milllimeters daily for as long as four to five years); a brief period during which hair growth ends, called *catagen*; and a "resting" phase called *telogen*, during which your hair remains in its follicle but does not grow.

Studies of normal, healthy scalps reveal that approximately 90 percent of the hairs on your scalp are anagen hairs, while 10 percent are in the telogen phase. The telogen, or resting phase, lasts for several months and ends when these hairs fall out or are pushed out by a new anagen hair. Resting hairs are called "club" hairs because of the bulbous, club-shaped thickening of the hair shaft at the scalp end of the hair. This thickening is not the "root" of the hair—a fear of many people who examine their falling hair. It is reassuring to know that club hairs are always being replaced by new anagen hairs. The average scalp sheds fifty to seventy-five hairs daily, so you will scarcely notice the loss. Usually only a few of these hairs are seen on your brush or comb, in the sink, or on the pillow, and your scalp hair will appear full and healthy.

Why Hair Falls Out

It frequently happens that a young woman enters a dermatologist's consulting room clutching to her bosom a small plastic bag filled with hair. She tearfully tells the physician that she is losing all her hair. The doctor examines the woman's scalp and tugs gently at her hair, pulling out several strands with ease. He examines the hair in the plastic bag and, like the hairs in his hand, most have whitish club-shaped swellings at the end of the hair shaft.

The dermatologist asks if she has a new baby. Startled, the woman admits she does. He assures her that her hair will soon stop falling out and will regrow normally in due time.

The fact is that childbirth is one of the most frequent causes of a temporary type of hair loss called *telogen effluvium*, a term that describes the rapid shedding of many hairs in the resting phase of the hair cycle. The hormonal changes associated with pregnancy alter the normal hair cycle by encouraging many hairs to continue to grow after their growth phase should have ended. Immediately after childbirth, when hormone levels drop, many of these hairs stop growing and enter the resting stage. They then undergo a normal shedding three to four months later, and many hairs are lost in a relatively short period of time. This rapid hair loss may continue for several months, but new hairs replace the lost ones, and sooner or later there is a return to a normal balance of growing and resting hairs.

Women who discontinue the use of birth control pills often experience a similar pattern of hair loss occurring three to four months after the last cycle of pills has been taken. In a sense, the female hormones in the pill mimic the hormone changes that are associated with pregnancy.

Certain diseases and physical stresses can similarly affect your hair cycle. For instance, in the days when bacterial pneumonia and typhoid fever caused sustained high fevers, a "postfebrile" form of hair loss was quite common. Today surgery, general anesthesia, or a successful "crash" diet with a thirty- to forty-pound weight loss are the physically stressful situations most likely to cause hair loss (sudden weight loss deprives your rapidly dividing hair cells of protein, thus interrupting your normal hair cycle). A severe emotional shock is often suggested as a cause of telogen hair loss, but it is difficult to prove that mental anguish alone can trigger a loss of hair.

If the physiological mechanism underlying this form of hair loss is understood, it is clear that no treatment is possible, or, for that matter, necessary. The physical stress that may have triggered your hair cycle problem occurred several months before the hair loss was apparent. The damage has not only been done, but has been corrected naturally by the time your hair is beginning to fall out in large numbers. As night follows day, your hair loss will come to an end, and new hairs will emerge to fill in the vacant follicles. The exceptions to this happy solution are the rare ongoing diseases and hormonal problems that must be corrected before the hair cycle returns to normal.

Many patients who experience this form of hair loss intellectually understand the nature of the problem but nevertheless demand some kind of treatment. They often ask for vitamins, massage, or ultraviolet light to hasten the return of their hair. The honest physician tells them to save their money. There is no hair-growing medicine that will hasten a return to a balanced hair cycle.

Treatment of Hair Loss

Some causes of hair loss are amenable to treatment. Your dandruff and itchy scalp are manifestations of seborrheic dermatitis, a condition that sometimes is associated with loss of hair. Appropriate treatment with medicated shampoo or scalp lotion will clear up the dermatitis and stop your hair from falling out. Your lost hair will regrow since the dermatitis does not cause any permanent damage to the hair follicle.

Other inflammations of the scalp such as psoriasis, eczema,

or infections are at times associated with an unpredictable and patchy hair loss. Treatment of the basic disorder will correct the altered environment of the scalp and encourage the hair to regrow. Occasionally, a severe inflammation or infection will irreparably damage some of the hair follicles to the extent that they become incapable of regenerating hair.

There are also several medications that cause a generalized but temporary loss of scalp hair. These medicines are used in the treatment of serious illnesses and the hair loss should be viewed as but a minor side effect. For example, drugs employed in the chemotherapy of cancer and leukemia can damage the sensitive hair cells in the same manner that they attack the tumor cells. If the hair cells are unable to grow and multiply in a normal fashion, the hair shaft becomes thin and fragile. Some of the most potent chemotherapeutic medications will stop hair growth completely, and profound hair loss may follow, resulting in total baldness. Reports suggest that the application of an icebag to the scalp during chemotherapy can minimize hair loss. Once the course of chemotherapy is terminated, the hair will regrow, but it will be months before recovery is complete.

Vitamin A is an example of a "medication" that can cause hair loss if amounts exceeding the daily requirements are ingested for a prolonged period, which should never be the case. A group of vitamin A–like drugs, the retinoids, occasionally have the same side effect. The hair grows back after the completion of a course of therapy with a retinoid.

Thyroid pills are often prescribed for the treatment of thinning hair on the chance that your hair loss is due to an underactive thyroid gland. If the functioning of your thyroid is in question, blood tests should be taken that give a clear indication of the gland's activity. Afterward, thyroid supplements may be prescribed. Thyroid tests are recommended for many individuals with persistent, unexplained hair loss, since this is one of the few ailments where diagnosis and treatment will correct the problem.

As mentioned earlier, iron deficiency is another correctable condition that is sometimes associated with falling hair. Women with anemia due to prolonged or heavy menstruation may experience an associated hair loss that can be corrected by treatment with iron pills or injections.

Baldness

Hair loss and baldness (*alopecia*) would seem to be a matter of cause and inevitable effect. Fortunately, this is not always the case. Although a separation of these two problems may be somewhat arbitrary, the previously discussed causes of hair loss rarely lead to the condition called *baldness*, which is defined as the state of the scalp when some portion of it is completely devoid of hair.

Male-Pattern Baldness

The common form of male baldness (*androgenetic alopecia*) evolves in a distinctive, easily recognizable pattern. In the earliest stages of baldness, there is a recession of the hairline in the front of the scalp by the temples. Although some degree of hair loss in this area is perfectly normal in young men, the change from what is considered a normal mature hairline to the early stages of male baldness is almost imperceptible.

As male baldness progresses, the frontal hairline recedes further and thinning occurs on the top of the scalp. Sooner or later, the thinning areas blend together and the familiar end result is a bald scalp with a circumferential fringe of hair.

There are three acknowledged factors that determine the occurrence and, to some extent, the severity of male baldness. First, a family history of baldness is an indication that the inherited tendency is present and can be passed on to subsequent generations. Baldness in male members of the maternal side of the family or in the father raises the odds of male-pattern alopecia in the male offspring.

Second, the presence of male hormones (androgens) is an essential factor in male-pattern hair loss. Male baldness does not occur before puberty, and males who have been castrated do not go bald.

Time is the third critical factor in male balding. The incidence of baldness among men increases with age; by age sixty, close to 80 percent of all Caucasian men are partially or completely bald. While black and Asian men are not immune to male-pattern baldness, the incidence is much less than in Caucasians.

Young men often become alarmed when they note a sudden thinning out in the characteristic male-pattern areas. They logically assume that, at the rate the hair loss is progressing, total baldness is inevitable at an early age. Although some concern is justifiable, the long-term prognosis is difficult to predict, because the hair loss associated with male baldness occurs at irregular intervals. Large amounts of hair may fall out over a period of months and then the hair loss may stop completely. The next flurry of hair loss may not occur for many more months, or even years. Furthermore, every hair that falls out is *not* a hair gone forever. Fallen hairs are replaced by new hairs, which tend to become smaller and thinner with each cycle of hair loss. This process may continue for years. The ultimate end stage is a smooth scalp with a scattering of light fuzz.

Women are not immune to the male form of baldness, which in most cases occurs after menopause, when there is a shift in the estrogen-to-androgen ratio. Young premenopausal women who develop a pronounced male-pattern baldness should be examined by a gynecologist and have appropriate tests performed to determine if they are producing abnormal amounts of androgen hormones.

Treatment

Minoxidil Until recently, no other group of cosmetically impaired people has been more taken advantage of by quacks and unethical cosmetologists than men and women with male-pattern baldness. This situation has changed, however, since the discovery of minoxidil. An oral medication developed in the 1970s to treat high blood pressure, minoxidil had the unpleasant side effect of growing superfluous hair (*hypertrichosis*) in patients who used it. This clinical observation led in time to the development of minoxidil as a scalp lotion for the treatment of male-pattern baldness.

In the initial studies of the drug, approximately one-third of balding men grew hair after applying a minoxidil lotion to the scalp twice daily for three to four months. Unfortunately, the hair growth occurred only at the top of the scalp but not in the frontal, receding hairline areas. Men with early baldness responded better than those with a well-established bald pate, and it appears that treatment must be continued indefinitely to maintain the new hair and prevent further hair loss—an expensive proposition, to say the least. It is not understood why minoxidil grows hair.

Minoxidil is the first hair-growing medication to undergo rigorous testing and to receive approval of the Food and Drug Administration (FDA), but it still must pass the test of time as well as widespread use by many people for ultimate public acceptance and approval. The discovery of minoxidil has also spawned a group of me-too hair-growth cosmetic lotions and creams on the market. But unlike minoxidil, these nonmedications have not been scientifically appraised, nor have they received the approval of the FDA, so there is no reason to expect that they will help at all.

In the future there may be even more effective minoxidil derivatives. Another avenue of hair research involves studying the local effects of anti-androgens, chemicals that may block the negative effects of androgen on the hair follicle. At the present time, successful results with these antihormones have not been reported.

Hair Implants Advanced male baldness can be alleviated by one of several cosmetic or reconstructive procedures. Artificial hairpieces, or hair weaving—the process of incorporating human hair into thinning areas of the scalp—will satisfy some, but many balding men seek a more permanent solution. The implantation of hairlike nylon filaments that are sutured or otherwise anchored into the scalp skin has been largely abandoned because of problems with infections or reactions to the foreign materials used in the procedure.

To date, the *hair transplant* technique is the most widely used and the most acceptable procedure for fighting hair loss. Grafts of normal hair-bearing scalp from the patient are transferred from the back of the head, where the scalp is not affected by baldness, to the frontal bald areas. This is accomplished by excising ¹/₁₆-inch circular areas of scalp skin with a round cutting instrument called a "punch." These circular areas of scalp skin are then placed into similar-sized holes from where sections of the bald scalp have been removed, thus establishing a new hairline, or filling in a thinned area. The hair removed from the back of the scalp does not grow back, but the scars can be camouflaged by permitting the hairs above the scar to grow long and to cover over the defect. The extent of baldness determines how many hair grafts are required to provide adequate covering. Usually, the transplantation is carried out in several operative sessions.

If everything goes well, side effects from this surgery should be relatively minor. There's overnight pain, temporary swelling that might appear after a day or two, and a sensation of numbness that could last for weeks or months until nerve endings regrow. More serious but rarer side effects include postoperative bleeding, which may require additional stitches, and infection, which is treated with antibiotics. There can also be a psychological burden: If the bald area is large, the healing and hair-growing process may be visible to the world.

Although it is difficult to generalize about cosmetic surgery, most people who have the hair transplants seem satisfied, if not ecstatic, with the results. The procedure is not a total solution, since only a thin hair covering is established, and repeated operations may be necessary as hair loss continues its march to the back of the scalp. Furthermore, many hair transplants can be recognized for what they are, which detracts from their value in providing a "natural" look. There's also considerable debate among dermatologists about whether hair transplants offer enough cosmetic improvement to be worth the time, cost, and discomfort.

Alopecia Areata

Alopecia areata is a localized area of baldness that develops rather suddenly on the scalp, beard area, eyebrows, or on any other area that bears hair. Your barber or hairdresser may be the first to perceive the bald spot and refer you for medical evaluation.

Although dermatologists recognize that this condition is a

distinct and separate form of baldness, they are unable to explain its cause. Traditionally, it's been suggested that alopecia areata follows an emotional or physical shock, although there is no scientific data to support this theory. More recently this type of hair loss has been viewed as an *autoimmune* response—a phenomenon where the body's immune cells assault the hair follicles for inexplicable reasons.

In some cases, where there are one or two small bare spots, the hair will grow back in months without treatment. When dermatologists are consulted, they often resort to the use of corticosteroids injected directly into the skin of the bald area. This form of treatment may be helpful to some patients with alopecia areata. Still, even though the cortisone-like drugs accelerate the growth of hair, the results of the treatment are often unpredictable and short-lived, for the new hair growth may suffer the same inexplicable tendency to fall out.

In severe cases, where there are multiple large bald spots that continue to expand, systemically administered corticosteroids might decelerate, if not arrest, continued hair loss. The side effects of these drugs, however, may limit their use (see pages 28–29).

Minoxidil lotion has been tried in treating alopecia areata, with only about 10 to 15 percent of users showing any regrowth of hair. This is not an impressive response rate since almost everything else that has been used to treat this condition does at least as well.

Sad to say, there are children and adults who lose all their scalp hair, and sometimes their body hair, from this mysterious disease. Complete and permanent hair regrowth is highly unlikely in these most severe forms of alopecia.

Traction Baldness

Hairstyling can be another form of hair trauma that can lead to hair breakage. Hairstyles such as a ponytail or a bun, which pull the hair tight, can cause a form of hair loss called *traction baldness*. Women can also suffer this form of baldness due to hair styling practices such as braiding or cornrowing. Hairs that are tightly wrapped around rollers night after night may suffer the same fate.

Treatment is simple: stop the form of hairstyling that is pulling on the hair, and wait for the lost hair to grow in again. If the particular styling process is continued for a long time, the hair loss may be permanent.

COSMETIC HAIR PROCEDURES

One of the paradoxes of modern hair care is that many of the cosmetic procedures that we use to beautify and improve the character of our hair can damage its structure. For example, in the case of hair dye, the chemical agent present in dark brown or black dye can cause allergic contact dermatitis. Since it is the scalp that suffers the brunt of the rash, however, damage to the hair is usually mild and rarely causes more than a temporary hair loss.

More often, hair damage occurs when the chemicals used in the dye process are detrimental to the protein that is the backbone of the hair. In order for a "permanent" dye to be fixed to the hair, it must penetrate and enter the heart of the hair shaft. This is accomplished by a chemical assault on the hair's outer surface that quite literally makes holes in the hair. Further structural damage occurs when the dye is chemically altered so that it remains bound to the internal hair protein. In some color changes it is cosmetically advantageous to remove the normal hair color before dye is applied, a process referred to as "stripping." The strong chemicals used to strip can further weaken the structural integrity of the hair.

If stripping and dyeing are repeated at regular intervals, the hair suffers cumulative damage, although it may take years before there are obvious signs of hair breakage. Tolerance to these procedures varies, and it is difficult to predict what type of hair is most vulnerable; much will depend upon the skill and care of the operator who lays on the dye and the other chemicals. No matter how carefully the procedure is carried out, however, the nature of the alteration is such that it is likely that some hairs will sooner or later break or fall out.

It is surprising that permanent waving doesn't lead to more frequent hair-loss problems. The chemicals used in perms rupture the hair proteins and then reassemble them in a new wave shape. It is reasonable to assume that the newly arranged protein is not as strong as was the original form. But the fact is that hair breakage is an uncommon side effect of the permanent—if it is performed in a careful manner by a skillful operator.

Regular Hair Care

These worst-case descriptions of cosmetic hair procedures should not leave you with the impression that modern hair care is a dangerous game to play. For most people, dyeing or styling of the hair does not cause perceptible damage. Furthermore, there are many other aspects of hair care that are both safe and helpful to the overall well-being of your hair.

Shampooing your hair with a soap shampoo at regular intervals is a pleasant and healthy procedure. Many youngsters shampoo daily and their hair and scalp are none the worse for it.

Hair sprays and conditioners are also usually well tolerated. Some after-shampoo rinses contain electrically charged chemicals that counteract the static electricity that makes hairs repel each other, thus eliminating the frizzy look. Other rinses merely deposit an oil on the hair that creates a sheen without producing a tacky feeling. These popular preparations are unlikely to be a source of hair or scalp problems.

For grooming thinning hair, you can use creams and gels containing a mixture of protein and oils that "build up" the remaining hairs. These products are not effective remedies for incipient baldness, but they are safe and rarely damage your hair.

The use of hand-held hair dryers is so prevalent today that we should know by now whether or not blow-drying is damaging to the hair. Since problems are rarely, if ever, seen by dermatologists, it seems that moderate use of the blow-dryer is harmless. However, prolonged or excessive heat applied to the hair *will* dry it out and make it susceptible to breakage.

The practice of applying a rinse or temporary dye that can be washed out with an ordinary shampoo is considerably safer than the use of a permanent dye. A rinse colors only the surface of the hair shaft and the chemical interaction is minimal and reversible. This method is not as satisfactory to people who prefer a longer-lasting hair color change, however.

EXCESS HAIR

Hypertrichosis is a condition of excessive facial or body hair in women. It is possible for men to be hypertrichotic, but more often than not they are just plain hirsute. Since the amount of body hair that is considered normal covers a wide range, depending upon racial and familial factors, it is often difficult for a physician to assess a complaint of excessive facial or body hair. Cultural and individual tastes further confuse the issue. Some women will raise a fuss about a few hairs on the chin, while others will ignore an obvious mustache.

Growth of body hair in both men and women is controlled by androgens (male hormones) produced by the sex glands as well as the adrenal glands. The amount of body hair depends upon the quantity of androgen produced, the duration of hair follicle exposure to these hormones, and the inherent sensitivity of the hair follicles to the androgens. It is perfectly normal for older women to grow some facial hair when the androgens activate hair follicles made sensitive by aging.

Many women who consult a dermatologist with a complaint of excessive body or facial hair turn out to have normal amounts of hair when their familial and racial backgrounds are taken into consideration. In many other women the parameters of normalcy might be debatable, but ultimately no hormonal imbalance or other explanation is found that would indicate that the condition is abnormal.

In a relatively small number of women, the appearance of new and excessive amounts of hair is due to some disease of the ovaries or adrenal glands that causes an overproduction of androgens. Since these hormones have a masculinizing effect, there may be other clues to these disorders, such as a receding scalp hairline (as in male baldness), an increase in the size of muscles, acne, irregularities of menstruation, and a deepening of the voice. Most of the diseases that cause excessive androgen production can be treated, and when treatment is successful, the hypertrichosis and other symptoms are partially reversible.

There are several medicines that can cause hypertrichosis. Cortisone-like drugs, used widely in the treatment of a variety of diseases, will cause an increase in facial hair and sometimes body hair if they are taken for prolonged periods. Minoxidil, used as an antihypertensive medication, and diphenylhydantoin, a medication prescribed for epilepsy and other forms of convulsions, have a similar side effect.

Removing Superfluous Hair

There is no completely satisfactory method of eliminating unwanted hair. All of the techniques that are currently available have their drawbacks, and the world eagerly awaits a simple, safe, and painless method of permanent hair removal.

The techniques, in order of simplicity and frequency of use, are: cutting, plucking, shaving, bleaching, chemical depilation, waxing, and electrolysis. At one time X-ray treatments were used by commercial hair-removal clinics. Only years later did it become apparent that this misuse of X rays had some disastrous, long-range effects. Many of the people who were initially satisfied with this treatment developed chronic skin disease (radiodermatitis), and ultimately developed skin cancers in those areas of the skin where the hair had been removed.

Cutting and shaving of the hair are safe and simple methods of hair removal that some people find unattractive because they leave a stubble. There is an often-repeated belief that shaving encourages the hair to grow more rapidly and coarsely. This is not the case; the hair shaft tapers as it grows out, and severing it at the skin level creates an impression that the newly emerging portion of the hair is thicker and darker than the tapered portion that has been removed.

Bleaching with inexpensive hydrogen peroxide or the more expensive cosmetic bleaching creams is simple and unlikely to cause skin irritation. The major drawback is that the bleached hair is still there and may be only partially disguised by the lightening process. Chemical depilatories are popular and leave a smooth, hairless skin surface by rupturing the strands of hair protein and breaking the hairs inside the hair follicle. Since the epidermis surrounding the hair is also made of similar protein, the depilitating agent may irritate the skin.

Hair can be extracted from the hair follicle by a process called *waxing*. This technique—which may be compared to the pulling of a tooth—is generally performed in beauty salons because it does require some finesse. There are, however, waxing kits available for home use. Either warm or cold wax in a semisoft condition is applied; as it hardens, it envelops the hair and, when removed, pulls the hairs out of their follicles. Waxing is a rather painful process, but at least the intervals between treatments are longer than with the other methods of temporary hair removal. Waxing can cause irritation, however, and you should follow the instructions on the kits carefully.

In electrolysis—the only permanent technique of hair removal—a fine needle is inserted into the hair follicle, and an electrical impulse is delivered to the sensitive hair bulb. The intention is to permanently destroy the growth center of the hair and thus prevent it from regrowing.

There are several drawbacks to electrical hair removal. It is not a home method, since it requires relatively expensive equipment and a licensed operator (electrologist) trained in the use of the apparatus. (The hair removal kits available for home use do not employ a true electrolytic means of destroying the hair follicle; regrowth of hairs after using these home methods is inevitable.) Furthermore, even the most skillful electrologist can have problems with this technique. If too much electrical stimulation is delivered to the root area, damage to the tissue around the hair follicle can cause scarring in the form of a permanent retraction or puckering of the hair follicle opening. At the other extreme, insufficient electrical damage will not destroy the root and regrowth of the hair will occur.

Since it is better to err on the side of understimulation, if fifty hairs are removed at a treatment session, it is likely that ten or even twenty will regrow. This can make for a prolonged and expensive hair removal experience. Nevertheless, it is the only method that will permanently eliminate hair, and you should consider it for limited areas of superfluous hair.

THE NAILS

Finger- and toenails probably represent an evolutionary digression from the more utilitarian claws of four-legged animals. It is even possible that on the step up the ladder of evolution, they will disappear altogether. This may be overstating the case against nails; they do provide some protection for the sensitive tips of the fingers and toes and are helpful in carrying out fingertip functions such as manipulating a button into a hole or picking up tiny objects.

Nails are made of keratin, the same resilient protein that covers the skin surface and that constitutes the greater portion of the hair. The nail plate originates from a growth area called the *matrix,* which is partially hidden by the skin covering the tops of the fingers and toes. If the matrix is injured or diseased, it alters the normal appearance of the nail plate. In fact, if the skin covering the matrix is inflamed, it will also affect the contour of the nail plate.

Less than one-third of the nail is covered by skin. The portion

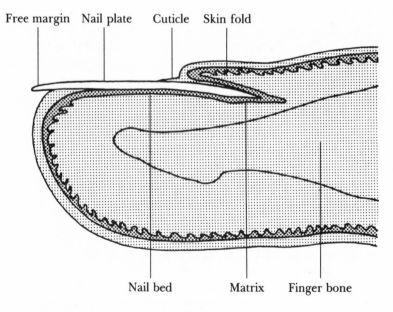

Figure 5. Cross section of a fingernail

of the nail peeping out from this partial covering is a pale, crescent-shaped area called the *lunula*. The lunula is part of the nail matrix, the portion of the nail that gives rise to the nail plate. The cuticle that surrounds the attached portion of the nail is really part of the skin and has nothing to do with the formation of the nail plate.

Considering that as an anatomic structure nails are not very important, they are subject to an amazing number of abnormalities, ranging from minor cosmetic changes to infections and structural irregularities.

Brittle Nails

Brittle nails rank with heartburn, insomnia, and aching feet as among the most common of medical complaints. A prevailing theory suggests that your nails become brittle when they lose water and quite literally dry out. Paradoxically, excessive exposure to soap and water also dehydrates the nail plate, as does a low-humidity environment.

If you suffer from brittle nails, you will not be helped by attempting to reverse the drying process through the avoidance of soap and water, or by the application of a lubricating ointment; however, since no other treatment is available, these maneuvers are worth a try. The old-fashioned gelatin treatment makes no sense at all, of course. Since your brittle nails have nothing to do with protein deficiency, ingesting a large dose of gelatin in a glass of tomato juice three times a day will not restore your nails to the desired degree of hardness.

Split Nails

Women often complain of the separation of the nail plate into layers at the unattached margin. Again, the cause is not clear, but drying out of the nails, in addition to exposure to household irritants, possibly contributes to the problem. It may help to protect your nails with rubber gloves during periods of household or industrial work. Like the brittle nail syndrome, your split nails are not a sign of nutritional deficiency, and consequently do not respond to vitamins or other dietary supplements.

Hangnails

Small hard projections of skin that have split away from the skin at the side of the nails are inappropriately called hangnails. They are seen most often in nail biters or in nervous individuals who manipulate and pick at the skin around the cuticle with another fingernail. Hangnails are significant only because they hurt, are unsightly, and allow bacteria to enter the broken skin, where it can cause a localized infection. Treatment is simple: Clip them off close to the skin's surface, and use an antibiotic ointment if the area is red and sore.

Nail Injuries

If you smash your thumbnail with a hammer, or get a fingernail caught in a door, the injury may cause blood to accumulate under the nail plate. If the accumulation of the blood causes severe pain, your dermatologist can quickly solve the problem. A steel safety pin or a similar sharp instrument is heated over a flame and then gently and painlessly used to burn a small hole in the middle of the damaged nail plate. The blood is able to seep out through the opening and the pain is relieved.

If the damage from a crush injury is severe, the nail plate will separate and fall off, but a new, healthy nail will usually replace it. If the nail remains attached, the plate may become discolored by trapped blood pigments that become incorporated into the nail, and it may be months before all traces of the injury grow out with the nail.

Nail Biting

Nail biting can sometimes result in hangnails, bacterial infections and warts, and deformity of the nail plate. There are no really successful methods of treatment, and the problem is often not solved until the nail biter decides that there are better ways of alleviating tension.

Another form of compulsive behavior is to push back the cuticle of the thumbnail with the adjacent forefinger nail. This repeated motion eventually damages the cuticle and the underlying nail matrix. The result is that the nail plate grows out with a linear irregularity extending from the cuticle to the free edge. Many people are unaware that they have this habit, and frequently visit their dermatologist to solicit treatment for a "nail fungus."

Spots, Lines, and Furrows

Pinhead-sized white spots and white lines are occasionally seen on otherwise healthy nails. Their cause is not known, but they are not a sign of any disease.

Longitudinal lines of varying degrees of prominence in the nail plate are so common as to be considered a normal finding. They become more apparent with age but, like white spots, are not associated with any disease. Another type of line, which is actually a depression or a furrow, runs across the nail from side to side. It may appear a few months after a serious operation or illness, either of which can temporarily arrest or slow the growth of the nail. These furrows ("beau's lines") grow out with the nail plate and disappear.

One of the most common causes of a longitudinal furrow or split in the nail is a blow or some other form of injury to the matrix, the growth plate under the skin. If the damage to the matrix is not repaired through the normal healing process, a scar results and the split becomes a permanent reminder of what otherwise might have been a rather trivial injury.

Ingrown Nails

Nails grow out and not in. The formation of what is mistakenly called an ingrown nail is due to pressure—often from ill-fitting shoes—that forces the side of the nail to dig into the skin. The area "ingrown" becomes sensitive, red, swollen, and infected.

The traditional methods used to treat ingrown nails are usually successful. But some people suffer a persistent or recurrent problem due to the shape of their toes and nails.

A conservative approach to treating ingrown nails is as follows:

1. Soak the affected foot in warm water and apply an antibiotic ointment to the inflamed area two to three times daily to eliminate the infection.

2. A doctor should remove any fragments of nail and clean away the dead or infected skin.

3. Place a wisp of cotton under the corner of the nail plate to slightly elevate it and to retract the nail plate from the area of "ingrowth."

4. Always cut the nail to form a straight edge with corners above the skin, rather than a gracefully curved free margin.

5. Wear loose-fitting shoes or the familiar mutilated shoe with a hole in it, and discard your old tight-fitting shoes.

If this program is adhered to with patience and consistency, you can avoid surgery. The alternative to this conservative approach is a partial or total "nailectomy." This may not always solve the problem unless a portion or all of the nail matrix is destroyed so that part or all of the nail does not regrow.

Diseases of the Nails

Bacterial and Fungal Infections Anyone who performs manual labor may suffer unnoticed scrapes and bruises of the skin around the nails. These minor nicks allow access to bacteria and the yeast fungus *Candida albicans,* which are the major causes of *paronychia,* or infection of the skin around the nail. When paronychial infections are caused by staphylococcus bacteria, you will experience redness, swelling, and severe pain. See a doctor, who will treat this bacterial infection by hot soaks, antibiotics, and sometimes a surgical incision of the infected area to permit the pus to escape.

In contrast, a yeast fungus causes a more low-grade, indolent infection. Although the skin around your nail is red and swollen, tenderness and pain are minimal, and pressure on the reddened area does not send you into paroxysms of pain.

The distinction between the two infections is important, because soaking a fungus-infected finger serves only to spread the infection. Moreover, the conventional antibiotics used to treat bacterial infections have absolutely no effect on fungus.

The correct treatment of the fungus paronychia is to keep your finger absolutely dry and to apply a medication containing nystatin, amphotericin B, miconazole, or one of the many other effective antifungal agents prescribed by your physician.

The yeast infection can spread from your skin and infect the adjacent portion of the nail plate. The infected nail then becomes discolored and irregularly ridged or otherwise deformed. The fungus can also approach from the front of the nail by entering through an area where there is a separation of the nail from the nail bed. The infection then spreads rapidly under the nail from the tip of the finger backward toward the cuticle. The treatment for a yeast fungus infection of the nail is basically the same as treatment for a skin infection. Keep the affected finger and nail scrupulously dry and apply an antifungal lotion or ointment around and under the nail plate. Although there are no internal medications for the treatment of minor yeast infections of the skin and the nails, more serious and persistent infections can be treated with the oral antifungal agent ketoconazole.

Another common skin fungus responsible for chronic athlete's foot can infect your toenails and fingernails as well. The infected skin on the side of your feet or palms of your hands appears thickened, red, and scaly. This may simply appear as dry skin, but the abnormal nails should draw attention to the correct diagnosis. Over a period of months or even years, the nails gradually become thickened and yellowish, and a white chalky material builds up under the nail plate.

The fungus that is responsible for these nail changes is not particularly contagious, though it is widely dispersed in the environment. Since exposure to the organism is inevitable, individual susceptibility determines whether you will acquire this infection or not.

Treatment for this form of nail fungus is protracted and not always successful. The locally applied fungus medications are ineffective because they cannot reach the critical area of fungus growth underneath the nail. The oral antifungal antibiotics griseofulvin and ketoconazole offer the only hope for a cure. These medicines reach the infected area through the bloodstream and prevent the fungus from extending deeper into the skin and nails. Since they stop fungus growth but do not kill the fungus, treatment must be continued until the infected nail has completely grown out, a process that takes six months for a fingernail and a year or longer for a toenail. Even if the antifungal antibiotics are taken religiously for many months, the cure rate is still on the low side. This fact, combined with the cost of a year or two of therapy, and the potential side effects of long-term use (headaches, stomach distress, allergic reactions) may discourage you from embarking on a course of treatment.

Effects of Disease on Nails Chronic skin diseases, such as psoriasis and atopic dermatitis (eczema), can cause small depressions ("pits") as well as other disfigurements, such as crumbling and discoloration of the nail. These problems are unsightly, but rarely cause any physical pain. While it is difficult to correct a nail that has been deformed in this way, painful corticosteroid injections into the skin overlying the nail matrix may create a smooth and healthy nail in a few individuals, but this is rarely worth the effort. Sound advice to the afflicted: treat the inflamed skin and be patient; the nails will often grow out in a normal fashion with time.

Nails and Subtle Symptoms Some unusual changes in your nails may be clues to internal illness. In diseases of the heart and lungs in which the blood carries insufficient amounts of oxygen, your nails may become enlarged and convexly curved, a condition called *clubbing*. Your nails also can lose their normal flat contour and become concave ("spoon nails"). This deformity is sometimes associated with iron deficiency anemia and can be corrected by restoring the iron levels in your blood to normal.

When the blood supply to your fingers or toes is reduced because of some circulatory disease, your nails become misshapen, split, and thinned out. These nails changes occur only when the circulatory problem has existed for a long period of time.

There are other subtle nail changes that a physician might detect in the course of a medical examination that can provide him or her with information about your general health.

Changes in the curvature of your nails may be a sign of thyroid disease; small points of bleeding underneath the nail plates—called *splinter hemorrhages*—are seen in infections of the heart (endocarditis) but also in healthy people who have sustained a minor injury to the nail plate. In severe kidney disease (uremia), your nails can take on a two-tone discoloration—half the nail plate white and the other half brown.

Wilson's disease, a rare condition that disturbs the function of the liver and brain, causes blue moons on your nails. Even medications taken in the past can leave their mark. Your nails may turn yellow from prolonged ingestion of tetracycline or slate blue from ingested medications containing silver.

Care of the Nails

Your nails are at their healthiest when they are just left alone, except, of course, for careful trimming of the nail plate at appropriate intervals. It is biting, pulling, overgrooming, or otherwise mutilating your nails that leads to infection and disfigurement. Manicuring is an acceptable form of nail care if it is not overdone; but repeatedly pushing back the cuticles will sooner or later lead to a space between the skin and the nail plate, which is a favorite site for an infection to develop.

It is safe to use nail polish, and unpleasant reactions to it are rare. Occasionally, women become allergic to one of the chemicals in nail polish; often it is formaldehyde resin that is added to the polish to make it adhere to the nail plate. In the "hypoallergenic" array of cosmetics, there are formaldehyde-free nail polishes, but they are not as adherent or resistant to wear and tear as the ordinary polishes. Women who become allergic to their nail polish develop rashes on the face, especially around the eyelids, and around other parts of the skin that they frequently or thoughtlessly touch. The skin around the nails rarely if ever shows signs of the allergy.

Nail hardeners do not do very much to truly harden nails, but some of them contain chemicals (including formaldehyde) that can cause the nail plate to separate from its bed, a process called *onycholysis*. The separation causes a large portion of the nail plate to appear as white as the normal, unattached free margin. Some pre-polish undercoats have been known to cause a similar problem of separation, as well as irritation of the skin around the nails.

Some nail biters often resort to artificial nails, but these are also a source of infection and irritation of the surrounding tissue; artificial nails often dehydrate, split, and chip the surface of the real nail plate. As such, they are not recommended. If, however, you insist on using artificial nails, remove them as soon as possible. Prolonged use can result in permanent damage to your natural nail.

8 THE LIPS AND MOUTH

Burning mouth, sore tongue, and cracked lips may not rank high on your list of serious complaints, but they are annoying symptoms. Your dentist is likely to claim that these non-teeth-related complaints are not in his domain and to defer to his medical colleagues. Your family physician may be sympathetic but is generally not well informed on this topic.

Enter the dermatologist. Over the years, skin doctors have acquired an interest in, and an understanding of, oral diseases, in part because other branches of medicine have neglected this area, but also because many of the skin diseases affect the oral cavity as well.

THE BURNING MOUTH SYNDROME

The tongue and the mucous membrane that lines the inside of your mouth are subject to soreness, burning, numbness, and other odd sensations that often defy diagnosis. The traditional, overused explanation for these complaints rarely stands up to close scrutiny. Nutritional deficiency is a favorite diagnosis, but usually there is no supporting evidence of dietary inadequacy or signs of vitamin deficiency (such as a red, smooth tongue or cracks and sores at the corners of the mouth). So it is not surprising that vitamins and other nutritional supplements can do little if anything to relieve your symptoms.

Allergic reactions or simple irritations from toothpastes, mouthwashes, lozenges, bridges, caps, dentures, denture cleaners, lipsticks, and even unusual foods are worth considering, even in the absence of any signs of inflammation inside the mouth. You can, of course, avoid almost everything that goes into the mouth on a trial basis to determine if your discomfort is related to contact irritation or allergy.

In most cases, though, your symptoms remain unexplained and a careful and thorough examination usually fails to turn up any signs of a serious disease. Luckily, the irritations are usually short-lived, and disappear in a few weeks.

Don't use mouthwashes, antibiotics, or other medications for a burning mouth when there are no signs of any disease that would respond to these treatments. If the mouth soreness is so severe as to interfere with eating, a physician can prescribe oral anesthetics such as dyclonine or Lidocaine that can be used as a mouthwash or spray before mealtimes.

WHITE SPOTS

The irritation caused by a sharp-edged tooth or dental filling is one of the most frequent causes of a white patch on the inside of your cheek. A similar whitish thickening is seen in "cheek biters" who nervously chew on the inside of their mouth.

Burns from medications, such as aspirin tablets that are retained in the mouth for local pain relief, or very hot foods (the famous "pizza burn") can cause similar white membranes to form that will disappear within a few days without any special treatment.

Multiple milky white spots scattered throughout the inside of your mouth can be a sign of infection with *Candida albicans,* the yeast fungus. This condition is also known as "thrush." Newborns can acquire this infection during passage through the birth canal. Adults who have taken large doses of antibiotics and those who are weakened by a debilitating illness are similarly vulnerable to oral candidiasis.

106

At one time, thrush was treated by painting the infected areas inside of the mouth with gentian violet, an antiseptic dye. This was both a messy and prolonged therapeutic process. Nystatin and other antifungal medications are currently used with far greater success. Nystatin is available in the form of a liquid suspension that can be deposited inside the mouth of an infant, or used as a mouthwash in older children and adults.

More persistent, lacy white patches are seen inside the mouth and on the tongue and lips in a skin disease called *lichen planus*. Usually a purplish, slightly scaly rash on your arms, legs, or lower back provides a clue to this mysterious but not serious illness. Lichen planus is not to be confused with *leukoplakia*, another oral, white-spot disease that is a more serious problem since these spots can be the precursor of cancer of the mouth. Leukoplakia appears in response to a persistent irritation of the mucous membrane. Heavy smoking is the primary irritant in most cases. Exposure to excessively hot foods, ill-fitting dentures, and chronic infection are often mentioned as potential causes of leukoplakia, but the fact remains that this condition is most often found among long-time heavy cigarette smokers. *Erythroplakia*—areas of reddened mucous membrane—are much less common than patches of leukoplakia. Erythroplakia usually indicates the presence of cancerous changes in the mouth and demands immediate attention and treatment.

If the leukoplakic patches fail to respond to a curtailment of smoking and the elimination of other sources of irritation, then the white patches must be removed surgically or destroyed by chemicals or by some other form of cauterization. Large doses of vitamin A, vitamin A lozenges, or topically applied retinoids (vitamin A–like drugs) are sometimes helpful in reducing the thickness or even eliminating leukoplakic patches. These medications are certainly worth a trial before you turn to surgery or other invasive forms of treatment.

SORES AND ULCERS

The canker sore is surely one of the most annoying and painful trivial ailments that plague humans. Canker sores are also called *aphthae,* meaning "ulcers," and an outbreak of multiple canker sores in the mouth is referred to as *aphthous stomatitis* (inflammation of the mouth).

Despite the fancy nomenclature, the cause of the all-too-common canker sore remains unknown. There are plenty of theories but no hard facts to support them. Emotional stress is a favorite explanation offered—again, with no evidence—by the very individuals who suffer episodic attacks of aphthae. Infection by the herpes simplex virus seems a credible explanation for those canker sores that occur simultaneously and are contiguous with fever blisters on the lips. Some canker sores do appear to respond to treatment with a tetracycline antibiotic suspension, suggesting that a bacteria (yet to be isolated) is the cause or contributes to the problem. Allergy to foods, such as nuts and spices, was once a popular causal theory. This explanation has been replaced by the more current concept of autoallergy, which implies that the canker sore is due to an inappropriate allergic reaction against one's own tissue, in this case the mucous membrane cells that line the mouth. The origin of this self-destructive form of allergy remains unexplained.

The treatment of canker sores is far from satisfactory. Many physicians have their pet remedies, but there is no consistent response to any medication. Tetracycline has its advocates; corticosteroids are favored by others. Some physicians prefer to cauterize the sores with silver nitrate—a painful treatment that does not speed up healing.

Most canker sores take two to three weeks to heal, regardless of medication or manipulation. During this time your doctor can prescribe oral suspensions of anesthetics (Lidocaine or dyclonine) or an antihistamine mouthwash that can provide some relief from discomfort.

There are two serious illnesses that are associated with blisters or ulcers inside the mouth. A condition called *erythema multiforme* occurs as an allergic response to a medication or infection, particularly with the herpes simplex virus. In addition to the painful sores inside the mouth and on the lips, varied (multiforme) skin rashes appear, including red blotchy spots, hives, and blisters. A serious and at times fatal form of the disease, the Stevens-Johnson syndrome, can be readily recognized by the presence of painful sores and scabs around the eyes and genital area as well as inside the mouth, accompanied by serious systemic symptoms such as a high fever and swelling of the joints.

Pemphigus is another rare but potentially lethal disease. In this condition a weakness in the binding together of cells in the epidermis causes the formation of superficial blisters. Frequently, the first signs of pemphigus are the presence of fragile blisters inside the mouth that break as soon as they form, creating shallow but painful ulcers that show little sign of healing. Sooner or later, blisters will form on the skin in a similar pattern of nonhealing sores, which will coalesce and lead to larger erosions that are similar to a bad skin burn. Although the cause of pemphigus remains obscure, it is considered to be one of the autoallergic diseases in which antibodies react against the epidermal cells. Both erythema multiforme and pemphigus are treated with the corticosteroids, or sometimes with other medications that suppress the body's immune response. In the case of pemphigus, these drugs have proven to be lifesaving.

PROBLEMS OF THE TONGUE

Inspection of the tongue has been a ritualistic part of the medical examination since the time of Hippocrates. Your tongue's appearance provides your physician with information about the hydration of your body, its nutritional status, and, to some diagnosticians, the general state of your health.

Although the tongue is subject to numerous ailments, two conditions are of interest because of their striking appearance and colorful names. "Black, hairy tongue" accurately describes a condition that often follows prolonged antibiotic usage, which encourages the fungus candida to grow on the tongue's surface. It is *not* to be confused with a tongue that has become rough-surfaced and discolored from a medication or too much licorice candy.

Most cases of black, hairy tongue respond poorly to treatment, but the tongue does return to a normal appearance in due time. The treatments that are often recommended are antifungal medications or peeling chemicals. These medicines can be applied or scrubbed into the areas of disease with a toothbrush.

The "geographic" tongue presents an equally striking appearance. In this tongue disease the normal fingerlike projections on the surface of the tongue disappear and smooth, red spots with whitish borders form. The spots slowly enlarge and coalesce, creating a maplike appearance that changes regularly, suggesting the other name for this condition, "wandering rash of the tongue."

The cause of this peculiar-patterned tongue is not known. It rarely produces any symptoms and invariably disappears without medical intervention. Most people with geographic tongue are content if they are told they don't have cancer and that their peculiar-looking tongue will one day regain its healthy appearance.

PROBLEMS OF THE LIPS

The lips, like the mouth and tongue, are also subject to several annoying but rarely serious ailments.

Chapped, Cracked, and Peeling Lips

Cracking and peeling lips, made worse by winter weather, are a common complaint. Cracked lips are often the fate of "lip lickers" who attempt to relieve dryness with a little saliva. Invariably, this makes matters worse since the evaporation of the moisture has an additional drying effect.

There is no commercial lip balm that will work a healing miracle. Most lip medications provide you with no more than a lubricating, water-retaining film. For this purpose petroleum jelly or comparable greasy ointments are as useful, if not aesthetically as pleasing, as many of the commercial lip balms.

If lip peeling occurs throughout the year, you should consider causes other than the winter wind. Allergic reactions to lipstick, mouthwash, dental cleansers, mentholated cigarettes, or food dyes can cause a low-grade irritation indistinguishable from simple chapping. In the elderly, years of sun exposure may lead to peeling and splitting of the lower lip, a sign of irreversible sun damage. Once established, this irritation is difficult to treat, but it certainly can be prevented with a little foresight by limiting your sun exposure and using a protective lipstick that contains PABA or one of the other chemical sunscreens.

Splits at the corner of the mouth occur in "droolers," where the facial contour or a dental problem permits saliva to accumulate in this area. Denture wearers are particularly prone to this condition when the dentures do not afford a smooth, even bite (the uneven bite is called a *malocclusion*). If this is the situation, mechanical adjustments of the dentures, or new dentures, will eliminate the irritation.

Since moist skin is the playground of candida albicans, an infection with this fungus may complicate the irritation at the corners of the mouth and require local treatment with nystatin or one of the other antifungal creams. Many physicians will needlessly prescribe vitamin B complex as part of their treatment, since a deficiency of this group of vitamins is responsible for soreness and a rash inside and around the mouth in rare cases of malnutrition.

Contagious Conditions Affecting the Lips

A number of infections that occur on and around the lips can be passed on to another person by direct contact. *Impetigo,* the bacterial skin infection, is particularly contagious. One moist, red, or yellow-crusted sore leads to another, and infection of family members through direct contact or by using a common towel is likely if care is not taken. Similarly, *herpes simplex* in the active blistering stage, whether as fever blisters, cold sores, or so-called sun poisoning, is infectious, particularly to children and others who have not been previously exposed to the virus and have not developed protective immunity.

Other sores occurring inside the mouth are painful and slow-healing, but not contagious to others. The once prevalent "trench mouth" is not an infectious condition, but rather a reflection of poor dental hygiene, malnutrition, and generally lowered resistance. Similarly, the ubiquitous canker sore is a disease that rarely affects more than one member of a family at a time.

Infectious mononucleosis, a systemic illness, is a viral infection of young people. It was once called the "kissing disease," but according to most studies this mode of contagion seems unlikely. The virus that causes AIDS can be found in saliva, but the spread to another through casual oral contact is thought to be unlikely. There is little doubt, however, that *viral hepatitis* and many of the viral respiratory infections are transmitted by contact with saliva or droplets of mucus. Furthermore, these viruses may remain in the secretions long after signs of liver or respiratory infection have disappeared. In general, there should be more concern about the *unseen* infectious agents present than about the more obvious sores and blisters that deter intimate contact with the infected person.

9 SKIN INFECTIONS AND SEXUALLY TRANSMITTED DISEASES

For some inexplicable reason, it is widely assumed outside of the medical profession that most skin disorders are infectious. This prejudice is so deeply ingrained that it is difficult to convince people that this is not the case. Most of us tolerate the person who coughs and sneezes bacteria or viral particles into the atmosphere, but shun the individual with a skin rash as if he or she were the proverbial leper.

The truth is that most skin diseases are not infectious, and even many of the true infections are not very contagious. Those that are can be avoided by using a few simple precautions on a routine basis—usually involving soap and water.

A number of these diseases are minor annoyances, but some can develop into more serious conditions if they are neglected or improperly treated. Skin infections are caused by bacteria, viruses, and fungi. This chapter covers the most common of these diseases, as well as the increasingly important group that is transmitted through sexual contact.

BACTERIAL INFECTIONS

Bacteria are microorganisms—once referred to as "germs"—that bridge the gap between plant and animal life. They are visible under an ordinary microscope, but not with the naked eye. There are many perfectly harmless bacteria that regularly reside on the skin surface and undoubtedly contribute to its general well-being. It is virtually impossible to eliminate these bacteria, even by the most stringent methods of washing and sterilization. Skin infections, however, occur when abnormal, disease-producing bacteria make their home on the skin surface or inside a hair follicle.

Folliculitis

If an infectious strain of the staphylococcus bacteria finds its way into the opening of a hair follicle, a small pus pimple with a red area around it appears on your skin. This form of bacterial folliculitis occurs frequently in men from the minor trauma associated with shaving. Once entrenched in one or two follicles, the bacteria spread with ease to the adjacent follicles and the entire beard area may become infected.

Your dermatologist will take into account the manner in which folliculitis spreads and is perpetuated. The following regimen is usually successful if you follow it for several weeks:

1. Before shaving, thoroughly wash your face with an antibacterial soap.

2. After shaving, apply an antibiotic lotion or cream to the infected areas and the adjacent hair follicles.

3. Keep the razor submerged in alcohol or another disinfectant between shaves. Avoid electric razors temporarily unless they can be satisfactorily disinfected by dipping only the head in alcohol.

4. Take an appropriate oral antibiotic such as penicillin, erythromycin, or cephalosporin for a period of one to two weeks. If the infection is very resistant to treatment, the dermatologist will usually culture an infected follicle and test the bacteria that grows on the culture in order to determine what antibiotics will be effective.

Boils

Painful, deep, red nodules develop when the staphylococcus bacteria infect the deepest portion of the hair follicle and the inflammation spreads into the surrounding skin. Boils can occur wherever there are hair follicles, but the back of the neck and axillary (underarm) areas are common sites of this type of infection.

A solitary boil that heals by itself is a rather common problem that is ignored by many people or treated with home remedies such as hot compresses and drawing salves. The boil will usually disappear through a process of shrinking and absorption, or it may come to a "head" and discharge a pus-filled core. Multiple boils or sequential boils that appear over weeks or months require treatment by a dermatologist with an appropriate oral antibiotic.

Boils occur in perfectly healthy people, but multiple or recurrent boils are always a warning that something may be wrong with your immune system's ability to combat bacterial infection. More often, you are immunologically intact, but the strain of staphylococcus bacteria is singularly virulent and difficult to eliminate. Even after the series of boils have healed, the staphylococcus may continue to hide inside your nose, in the groin area, and under your arms. Individuals who thus become staph carriers transmit the infectious bacteria to others, and are themselves likely to experience recurrent attacks of boils over a period of months or years.

A prolonged course of treatment with a staph-killing antibiotic carefully chosen by a dermatologist, plus good general hygiene, is required to eliminate the carrier state. External treatment should include a daily bath with an antiseptic soap and frequent applications of antibiotic cream inside the nose and to the skin areas where the staph may reside.

For many years, physicians have treated patients suffering from resistant boils with vaccines made from bacteria that was cultured from the infected skin. But it is unreasonable to believe that a vaccine would stimulate an immune response when the same bacteria living deep in the skin fails to do so. Most physicians have discarded this approach because it is both illogical and ineffective.

Erysipelas

At one time, the skin infection *erysipelas*, which is caused by the streptococcus bacteria, was referred to as St. Anthony's fire.

The rash of erysipelas *is* a fiery red, tense swelling of the skin that spreads inexorably across the face or up the leg, until your body defenses or antibiotic treatment stops its progress.

In most cases, a small crack in the skin around the ears or between the toes serves as the entry point for the bacteria. Once inside the skin, chemicals released by the streptococcus bacteria facilitate the rapid spread of the infection.

The rash of erysipelas is usually preceded by fever, chills, muscle pains, and headache. The rash that follows is often mistakenly considered to be unrelated to these premonitory symptoms, and suggests two illnesses: perhaps a viral illness or a rash of unknown cause. This erroneous double diagnosis delays the start of a much-needed antibiotic treatment.

The treatment of erysipelas with penicillin produces one of the most dramatic therapeutic responses in all of medicine. Within a matter of a few hours, the fever drops to normal levels and the other symptoms quickly subside. The rash of erysipelas, however, may take a number of days to disappear completely.

VIRAL INFECTIONS

In contrast to bacteria, viruses are much smaller infectious particles that can cause disease only when they find their way inside a living cell. Viruses can enter your skin cells in two ways: through the bloodstream, as in the case of systemic viral infections such as measles and chicken pox, or directly from the external environment, as in the case of localized viral infections such as warts or herpes simplex.

Herpes Simplex

Fever blisters, sun blisters, and cold sores are familiar terms used to describe recurrent skin infections caused by the herpes simplex virus. Although almost everybody will suffer from one infection from this virus in childhood, 15 percent of the population will have a more permanent relationship with the virus, and will suffer from recurrent bouts of infection. In these individuals, the herpes virus may remain dormant in the body for months or years but, sooner or later, it will recur. In addition to sun exposure or fever, there are other factors that can trigger a herpes episode—illness, emotional stress, medications, and menstruation are some common causes.

The herpes rash consists of one or several clusters of small blisters that appear on an area of the skin that has already become swollen and red. The blisters often turn into pustules before they crust over and heal—a process that usually takes one week. Recurrent herpes is usually seen on the face and around the mouth, but any part of the skin of the upper body is susceptible. Most people who experience recurrent attacks of herpes are inconvenienced by the appearance of the rash and suffer some discomfort; only a very few are incapacitated by fever or other systemic symptoms.

The drug that is most often used to treat the first (usually the most severe) attack of herpes is an antiviral agent called acyclovir, which is marketed both as an ointment and as an oral tablet. This medication is recommended by the manufacturer for the treatment of herpes infections of the genital area, but many physicians use it for nongenital herpes as well. The value of acyclovir in recurrent attacks of both genital and nongenital herpes is not as clear-cut, but it is still widely used since no other specific remedies are available. Some patients who have frequent, severe episodes of recurrent herpes take acyclovir orally each day as a preventive measure in the hope of decreasing or stopping the herpes episodes. At this time, there are no known side effects of acyclovir, either in topical or oral form.

Many genital and nongenital herpes sufferers are not impressed with acyclovir in either ointment or oral form. They tend to rely on the old therapeutic standbys, which include compresses, antibiotic ointments to prevent superimposed bacterial infections, and various other over-the-counter products that may or may not dry up the blisters faster than Mother Nature.

Shingles

Unlike recurrent herpes simplex, a *herpes zoster,* or shingles, infection rarely occurs more than once in a lifetime. The virus responsible for shingles is the same virus that causes chicken

117

pox (varicella). Virologists believe that, after a person recovers from chicken pox in childhood, the virus remains in the body confined to a spinal nerve root. Years later it reappears, taking the form of a localized rash that breaks out on an area of skin that receives its nerve supply from a single spinal nerve. Shingles can occur at all ages, but it's much more common in late adult life.

Shingles is often preceded by pain, tingling, or pins-and-needles sensations in the affected area. These symptoms of neuritis (inflammation of a nerve) can persist throughout the attack of shingles, which lasts for two to three weeks. Sometimes, the pain continues long after the rash has healed, an unpleasant turn of events that is referred to as "postherpetic neuralgia."

Like herpes simplex, the shingles rash consists of several areas of skin that are red and swollen and covered with clusters of blisters. These blistering areas follow the path of a spinal nerve on one side of the body, most frequently on the torso or face.

There are two common misconceptions about this viral illness. Many patients, when informed they have shingles, believe that it is due to "nerves." Although a nerve is infected, in no way is this disease related to "nerves" in the emotional or psychiatric sense. A second misconception is that shingles is a potentially fatal disease if the rash spreads and completely encircles the body. This never happens. Although an attack of shingles can be extremely painful, it is not a serious ailment for people in good health. Individuals whose immune response to the virus is impaired by some other illness may experience complications due to the spread of the infection to the lungs or central nervous system.

Dermatologists usually treat the shingles rash initially with compresses to dry up the blisters, and apply lotions or salves to relieve the pain and to prevent bacterial infection. A short course of oral corticosteroids, if given early enough, may prevent the often protracted postherpetic pain that sometimes occurs in chronically ill or elderly people. Acyclovir capsules, given in large doses, will decrease the severity of a shingles attack, if treatment is started within several days of the onset of the rash.

Warts

The ordinary wart, *verruca vulgaris,* proves conclusively that an infectious virus can cause the growth of a benign tumor. Warts can be distinguished from other skin growths by their appearance. They are irregular, rough-surfaced nodules, with many small capillaries that appear as black dots that bleed easily if the wart is cut or traumatized.

Warts can thrive on any part of the skin surface, but the greatest number of warts occur on your hands and on the soles of your feet, where they are called *plantar warts.* Although warts can be spread from person to person, more often infected individuals reinfect themselves, as in the case of children who spread hand warts to their lips and face by chewing on their cuticles and fingernails.

The treatment of warts can be a lesson on the more mysterious side of medicine. Warts behave in very strange ways. Within two years from the time they first appear, 50 percent of all warts will disappear without any treatment, probably due to the development of an immunity to the virus. But it is also well known that warts may respond to "therapeutic" applications of raw potatoes, to hypnosis, and to positive suggestion, such as "your warts will disappear at midnight on the fourteenth of February." Physicians who have seen these remarkable events take place shake their collective heads in bewilderment. It may be pure coincidence that warts disappear in this manner, or perhaps the particular viral infectious disease does really respond to hypnosis and other forms of suggestion. Then again, these events may simply be related to immune changes in the body. The controversy continues.

A more conventional approach to the treatment of these nuisance growths relies on the removal or destruction of the wart tissue by a dermatologist using surgery, freezing, or the application of chemicals such as salicylic acid, trichloroacetic acid, or formaldehyde. Regardless of the choice of treatment, warts often regrow because the infectious virus remains in your skin even though the wart tissue has been removed. As with most other viral illnesses, the ultimate successful treatment of warts will more than likely be in the form of a vaccine that provides

119

children and adults with an immunity to this annoying, infectious disease.

FUNGAL INFECTIONS

For the layperson, the word *fungus* is often considered to be synonymous with skin rash. This misconception may well arise from the erroneous idea that most skin diseases are infectious. Although fungus can be contagious, it is not the epidemic or public health problem that many people think it is.

A fungus is a form of plant life. Species of fungus can range in size from microscopic single-cell forms to complex plants such as the edible mushroom. Although there are thousands of different species of fungus, only a handful are capable of causing skin diseases in human beings.

Ringworm

The term *ringworm* is used to describe infections of the skin that are caused by a number of different species of fungus. The name is misleading, since there is no "worm" involved in this infection, and the rash is not always in the shape of a ring.

Ringworm fungi live on the superficial, keratinized portion of the skin, nails, and hair, and infection of all three areas by the fungi can occur. Some common forms of this fungus tend to infect specific areas of the body, giving rise to such popular terms as *athlete's foot* (characterized by itching and scaling between the toes) and *jock itch* (an uncomfortable groin rash) for similar fungal infections.

A typical case of ringworm is easy to identify. Whether ring-shaped or not, the infected, red, scaly skin is sharply separated from the healthy skin by an elevated, rounded border. When the fungus attacks the scalp, there are round, scaly patches formed in areas that may eventually become bald, or at least show obvious signs of hair loss or breakage. Nails infected with ringworm fungus grow out thickened, misshapen, and discolored.

A diagnosis of fungus infection such as ringworm can be confirmed by scraping some skin cells from the suspicious rash and examining this material under a microscope for signs of the fungus. For further identification of the particular species, the skin scrapings can be placed in a culture medium, which will encourage the fungus to grow like a plant in a week or two for ready identification.

There are many medications available to treat fungus infections, including some excellent over-the-counter products. Nonprescription antifungal creams containing the chemicals miconazole, tolnaftate, or undecylenic acid are better-than-average treatments that rarely irritate the skin. The list of prescription medications for the problem grows longer each year. At the top of the list are econazole, ketoconazole, and clotrimazole.

Griseofulvin, an antifungal pill, is prescribed in cases of severe or extensive skin infections, or when the nails and scalp are involved. Prior to the discovery of this medication thirty years ago, ringworm of the scalp was very difficult to cure, and in many instances the fungus went unchecked until children "outgrew" the condition at puberty. Griseofulvin pills, taken for several weeks to a few months, will eliminate almost all skin and scalp infections. (Nail infections, however, require longer treatment, and permanent and complete cures of toenail infections are rare.) Griseofulvin is considered to be a relatively safe medication, even if months of treatment are necessary. The most common side effects are headache, stomach distress, and occasional allergic reactions, which all rapidly subside when the medication is discontinued. Ketoconazole is a newer oral antifungal medication that is about as effective as griseofulvin, although patients who are taking this drug must be monitored for possible liver toxicity.

Yeast Infections

The variety of external infections produced by the yeast fungus *Candida albicans* is quite remarkable. These include: sores at the corners of the mouth, swelling and redness of the skin around the fingernails, separation of the nail plate, white patches on the cheeks inside of the mouth, vaginal discharge, and a variety of moist, red rashes on the body. Although *Candida albicans* is widespread in the environment, increased susceptibility to the fungus appears to be the critical factor in many infections. The candida-prone group includes diabetics, individuals afflicted with other endocrine gland disorders, and diaper wearers, both young and old. Women who take tetracycline or birth control medication are also more susceptible to vaginal infections from this fungus. And since the fungus gravitates to areas of the body that are moist, obese people who perspire excessively are apt to acquire the infection under the arms, or in other areas where skin surfaces touch and the normal drying effect of evaporation is lacking.

A wide selection of medications is available that can be used to treat candida skin infections. Nystatin, miconazole, ketoconazole, and amphotericin B are popular remedies that can be prescribed for external application in the form of ointments, lotions, powders, or vaginal inserts. Nystatin can be taken orally; although it is not absorbed into the body from the intestinal tract, it will kill the fungus inside the lower bowel and thus eradicate this source of repeated skin and vaginal yeast infections.

Tinea Versicolor

A fungus with the euphonious name *tinea versicolor* has the distinction of causing the most common superficial infection, a rash that is easily recognizable as flat, brown, scaly patches on your chest, back, and upper arms. Sometimes the fungus de-pigments or lightens the infected skin, which makes the surrounding healthy skin appear contrastingly darker. This condition is particularly apparent in the summertime.

Tinea versicolor is a harmless infection. It rarely causes itching or other symptoms, and usually people seek medical attention only for cosmetic reasons.

There are several medications that will temporarily eradicate the scaly patches, but the infection can recur. At one time, a favorite prescribed remedy was for the patient to scrub his or her skin with a concentrated solution of sodium hyposulfate (a preparation that photography buffs will recognize as "hypo"). Better results are now achieved with a prescription for the chemical selenium sulfide in a shampoo vehicle, which is applied to the infected skin for 15 minutes and then washed off. Continue this treatment once daily for at least 4 to 6 weeks. Some of the antifungal lotions that are used to treat ringworm and candida infections also can be used to treat tinea versicolor, but the extent of the rash and the necessity of prolonged treatment makes cost a consideration.

OTHER INFECTIOUS DISEASES

Lyme disease, Rocky Mountain spotted fever, and toxic shock syndrome are not, strictly speaking, skin disorders. But since it often happens that a typical skin rash is the first symptom of these illnesses, they are included in this chapter.

Lyme Disease

In 1976 a small epidemic of new arthritis cases in the town of Lyme, Connecticut, led to the discovery of this new disease. Lyme disease is caused by a spirochete, a microbe that is transmitted to human beings by ticks. Adult ticks feed and mate on deer, then drop off to lay eggs. The eggs hatch into tiny deer-tick larvae, which contract the infection by feeding on mice, the primary carriers of the Lyme-disease spirochete. The larvae eventually molt into infected "nymphs," an adolescent stage that poses the chief threat to humans. Ninety percent of the cases of Lyme disease have occurred in eight states: California, Connecticut, Massachusetts, Minnesota, New Jersey, New York, Rhode Island, and Wisconsin. Lyme disease is clearly a summer disease, with about 90 percent of all cases occurring from early June through September.

The earliest sign of Lyme disease is an unusual rash at the site of the tick bite. Seventy-five percent of people infected will develop a red mark that spreads out to form a large ring, two to three inches in diameter. As the margin of the ring advances,

123

the central portion clears, creating a bull's-eye-like pattern. About half of the individuals with the large circular rash will develop multiple smaller spots scattered over the body. The skin rash of Lyme disease persists for three to four weeks and then disappears, even without treatment.

Other signs of infection are usually noted at the time of the rash. These include fever, headache, muscle pains, sore throat, and swollen glands. The more serious complications of the infection—neurological problems, heart disease, and arthritis—may not become apparent for weeks or months. Early treatment by a physician with appropriate antibiotics such as tetracycline or penicillin not only relieves the early symptoms but, more important, prevents the late complications. Since a blood test identifying the infection takes several weeks to become positive, it is reasonable for a physician to start treatment immediately if there is a suggestive history of tick exposure and if the characteristic rash is present.

Tick Removal A good tick-removal technique should work fast, getting the tick off before it's had time to inject its spirochetes into your body. (The mouth parts that penetrate the skin don't harbor spirochetes.) Research suggests that you have a grace period of at least a few hours from the time of the bite—so the sooner you remove the tick, the better.

Suffocating the tick with Vaseline, butter, or the like is largely ineffective. Gasoline, kerosene, and hot matches also work slowly if at all. Moreover, these all irritate the tick and may actually provoke it to release spirochetes into the skin.

The experts say there's only one good way to remove a tick, and that's to pull it out with tweezers or small forceps. Grasp the tick as close as possible to its mouth—the part sticking into the skin. Then, without jerking, pull it upward steadily. Don't worry about pulling out a little skin in the process.

The best tool for the job is a thin, curved forceps, available from surgical-supply stores and pharmacies. It's ideal for gripping the tick close to the skin and avoiding its bloated abdomen, which can act like a syringe if you squeeze it.

After removing the tick, disinfect the bite with rubbing alcohol or iodine. Don't handle the tick—dispose of it in alcohol or flush it down the drain. Check the bite occasionally for at

124

least two weeks to see if a rash forms. If it does, you've been infected and should seek treatment promptly.

Tips and Cautions In areas where tick-borne disease exists, it makes sense to take certain precautions—whether hiking in the woods or just strolling in the yard.

- Don't go out barefoot or in open sandals, and wear long pants. Cinching pants at the ankle or tucking them into boots or socks gives added protection.
- Wear light-colored clothing outdoors (it makes ticks easier to spot) and check your clothes every so often. Be especially careful in terrain with tall grass, bushes, or woods.
- Use a tick repellent, especially if you spend a lot of time outdoors.
- With children, start a bedtime check for ticks from about mid-April through September. Children are at a special risk because they spend so much time outside.
- Check pets for ticks. If a pet brings ticks inside, you can get infected without ever leaving the house.
- Know what to look for when making a tick check. A biting deer tick rarely hurts enough to draw your attention. To find one, you'll have to look for it—especially the tiny deer-tick nymph, which is smaller than a sesame seed. A nymph that's been attached to the skin for several hours looks like a blood blister with legs.

Rocky Mountain Spotted Fever

Rocky Mountain spotted fever is another tick-borne infection seen throughout the United States, with the highest incidence in the southern and western states. The ticks that spread the disease, the so-called wood tick and dog tick, carry infectious organisms called *Rickettsia*. Rickettsia differ from bacteria in that they can only survive inside a living cell. The rickettsial diseases include a chicken pox–like illness called *rickettsialpox* and typhus, an illness that throughout history has decimated the population of Europe and Asia with plaguelike epidemics.

The incubation period for Rocky Mountain spotted fever is three to four days following the tick bite. Actually only about two-thirds of infected individuals are aware that they have been bitten. The early symptoms of the infection are fever, severe headache and muscle pains, and nausea and vomiting. On the third or fourth day of the illness small, flat pink spots appear on the wrist and ankles and then on the palms and soles. The rash becomes reddish and the spots elevated as it gradually spreads up the arms and legs to the face and torso. After a few days the red spots become black and blue due to blood leaking out of the capillaries that have been damaged by the infection. The loss of blood and fluids throughout the body can cause shock and death.

Treatment Once the diagnosis is suspected, it is imperative to start treatment immediately. The antibiotics tetracycline and chloramphenicol are effective against rickettsia, and a good response to this treatment is usually evident within twenty-four hours.

Toxic Shock Syndrome

An infection with certain strains of staphylococcus bacteria is responsible for this acute febrile illness, which first shows up as a fever with an accompanying rash, often on the palms of the hands. These bacteria produce a chemical toxin that causes a rash in much the same way that the toxin made by streptococci causes the rash of scarlet fever.

In addition to the rash and fever, there may be a reddened swollen tongue, vomiting and diarrhea, and a shocklike condition. To date, a great majority of these toxic shock cases have been traced to the use of super-absorbing vaginal tampons.

Treatment Treatment consists of hospitalization to replace fluids, and the administration of a form of penicillin that will kill the staphylococci.

SEXUALLY TRANSMITTED DISEASES

Sexually transmitted diseases (STDs) include many more conditions than just syphilis and gonorrhea. A wide range of serious and not-so-serious diseases, transmitted through intimate body contact, come under this category.

Because many of these conditions first begin with a rash or some other type of skin manifestation, it is important that people recognize the symptoms promptly, in order to seek medical help for themselves and to avoid spreading the disease to others.

In this chapter we will consider the common forms of sexually transmitted diseases. In terms of prevention, there is no absolutely guaranteed way to avoid every form of a sex-related illness, except for complete abstinence from sexual contact—a remedy that is not practical or desirable for many people. The only other means of preventing the spread of these diseases is using caution when selecting a sexual partner, and the routine use of barrier methods of contraception, such as a condom.

Pubic Lice

A louse is a small, barely visible insect with a head, body, and six legs. Lice infest human beings and obtain their nourishment by attaching their mouths to the skin and ingesting blood. *Pediculus hominus pubis,* or *crabs,* is a distinct species of lice that makes its home in the hairs of the pubic area—the upper thighs, abdomen, and occasionally under the arms and on the eyelids. The lice reproduce by laying eggs (nits) that become attached to the hairs close to the skin surface.

Crab lice are usually acquired through intimate contact with a person who is infested. A long-standing debate continues about the possibility of contracting pubic lice from a source such as a toilet seat. In fact, the crab louse can survive a day or two off of the human body, which makes infection from bedclothes or other nonliving carriers a possibility.

Many patients suffer the intense itching produced by pubic lice for weeks or months simply because they fail to recognize the telltale signs of infestation—the presence of nits on hairs or the adult lice on the skin. Once the diagnosis has been made, however, treatment is relatively simple. There are several chemicals that kill the louse on contact. The most widely used is lindane (gamma benzene hexachloride), which is applied to the infested area following a bath. Twelve to twenty-four hours later, the medication is removed by another bath. At the same time, clothing and bedding are laundered or dry-cleaned, and all persons who have been intimate with the infected person are treated to prevent reinfection.

Genital Herpes Simplex

The herpes simplex virus (discussed on page 116) can also be sexually transmitted. The first attack of infection with the genital form of herpes simplex can be a highly uncomfortable experience for a woman, who may contract the infection from a sexual partner. The swelling and ulceration of the skin and mucous membrane in the genital region can cause severe pain that may last for several weeks. The first episode in males may be severe, but is usually not as incapacitating as it is in women.

The first attack of herpes typically begins within a few days after exposure to an infected person. Sometimes a newly infected person may feel burning or a pins-and-needles sensation before the outbreak; small blisters then appear on the labia, vagina, and cervix of women, and on the penis and scrotum of men. The blisters eventually break and form painful sores, which take two to three weeks to heal.

Treatment A woman newly afflicted with genital herpes may find some relief from warm "sitz baths" (sitting in a tub of warm water), from the use of a prescribed local anesthetic ointment (preferably lidocaine, which does not cause allergic contact dermatitis as do some other "caine"-type ointments), and from painkillers taken orally.

For both sexes, a prompt course of the antiviral agent acyclovir may shorten the first episode of the virus.

Recurrent genital herpes As in herpes simplex infections located elsewhere on the body, genital herpes is a recurrent problem in a minority of individuals who experience a first attack. These recurrent attacks may be triggered by any number of factors, including nervous tension, a febrile illness, or sexual activity. Fortunately, in most cases the recurrences become fewer and less severe as time goes by. A course of treatment with oral acyclovir, if administered within forty-eight hours of the onset of the recurrent attack, may shorten the duration of the infection.

In men recurrent genital herpes is an unpleasant experience that may lead to a temporary life of celibacy. In women, however, the herpes infection may have graver consequences. Statistical evidence suggests that this virus may play a role in the development of cancer of the cervix. Although a causal relationship is by no means clearly established, it is recommended that women who have had the herpes virus in the genital area be checked regularly by a gynecologist.

If a pregnant woman has had genital herpes, she should inform her physician of this fact. Although a past history of genital herpes does not harm the developing fetus, there is a possibility that an outbreak at the time of delivery might expose the baby to the virus. A herpes infection in a newborn is a serious matter, and can result in mental retardation, blindness, and neurological problems. In the case of a herpes flare-up, the delivery will be made by cesarian section, to avoid any chance of infection to the baby.

Many patients with recurrent genital herpes seek advice about the infectiousness of their sores. There is little doubt that the disease can be passed on to a sexual partner when there are actual blisters or a healing erosion on the skin. What is not so clear is the risk of contagion *before* the eruption, and *after* it heals. It is known that some individuals continue to shed the virus for days to weeks after the skin has healed. Clearly, the use of condoms and spermicidal foams (many of which are also viricidal) is indicated for patients with recurrent genital herpes.

Ironically, the panic produced by herpes in the 1970s has been superseded by concern about a far more serious disease, AIDS. This concern is changing sexual behavior in a way that will ultimately decrease the incidence of new cases of genital herpes in the future, although it is still widespread today.

Molluscum Contagiosum

Once almost exclusively a disease of children, the molluscum virus has left the classroom and found its way into the bedroom. The virus in adults is often spread through sexual contact, and the infectious lesions appear as smooth, rounded, pinhead- to raisin-sized bumps on the skin of the lower abdomen, thighs, and genital area. The infection is often ignored when there are only one or two molluscum papules present. But if this is left untreated, it may lead to dozens of new lesions spreading to other areas of the body, so a dermatologist should be consulted immediately.

Treatment The quickest and best way of eliminating molluscum growths is for the physician to scrape them off with a skin curette (a loop-shaped instrument with a cutting edge) after first freezing the skin with ethyl chloride to provide anesthesia. Since there is much less trauma involved in removing two molluscum growths rather than thirty-two, individuals with this infection are well advised to obtain treatment as soon as they recognize that the disease is present. Destroying the molluscum growths by freezing or chemicals are two other therapeutic methods that might be more suitable for children who are infected with the disease.

Venereal Warts

In adults, warts in the genital or perianal skin area are usually contracted through sexual contact. This is generally not the case in children, who transmit the wart virus from their infected fingers to the genital area. Venereal warts are very infectious and multiply in the moist environment of the genital and perianal skin area. No matter what treatment method is selected, the rate of recurrence after apparently successful therapy is discouragingly high. Since surgical removal is not recommended for these delicate parts of the body, other forms of therapy are preferred: the application of podophyllin or other chemicals, cryosurgery (freezing), or electrosurgery.

Syphilis

At one time, syphilis was the most dreaded of all infectious diseases. With the discovery of penicillin, fear of this illness has been replaced by a complacency that is not warranted. Syphilis still remains a serious and prevalent public health problem in many areas of the United States.

Syphilis is diagnosed by various blood tests. Once the diagnosis has been established, treatment with penicillin is curative in all cases, since the syphilis germ, *Treponema pallidum,* is universally sensitive to this antibiotic. In fact, it has been suggested that if every human being in the world were given penicillin at the same time, syphilis could be forever eliminated, since it is carried and transmitted only by human beings.

The study and treatment of syphilis fell into the hands of dermatologists mainly because all stages of the disease present prominent skin abnormalities. The *chancre,* a painless sore that appears where the syphilis germ has penetrated the skin, is the first sign of infection. Since syphilis is a sexually transmitted disease, most chancres will occur in the genital area, but chancres around the mouth and other parts of the body are common, depending upon individual sexual practices. The chancre develops about three weeks after contact with a person who has the infection. Even if it is ignored and goes untreated, it will heal spontaneously within six weeks.

When the chancre disappears, the infected individual will have entered the secondary stage of the disease, during which there may be a variety of symptoms, such as skin rashes, swollen glands, and fever. But even these symptoms will subside without any treatment. The infection may then remain dormant, hidden in the body for many years, before it again shows itself, reappearing as an inflammation of almost any organ of the body. At any stage of the disease, treatment with penicillin will stop the progress of the infection, but will not cure the body of the serious consequences from the long-term infection, sometimes including severe tremors or dementia.

Treating syphilis during pregnancy is particularly important because the infection can be transmitted to the fetus through the mother's blood. Infection of the fetus can result in miscarriage or produce a newborn with an active syphilitic infection (congenital syphilis).

Since syphilis can be diagnosed by a blood test any time after the beginning of the secondary stage, it is possible to identify and treat even infected individuals who do not show any outward symptoms of the disease. The premarital or preemployment blood tests routinely used in most states effectively screen thousands of people for the infection each year. Although this is a worthwhile practice, it does create some problems since the screening blood tests are very sensitive and sometimes show positive results in people who do not have the disease; a "false positive" test for syphilis can also occur in association with other illnesses ranging from minor viral infections to arthritis and cancer.

Most physicians are familiar with the "false positive" phenomenon, and will never assume that a patient with a positive blood test actually has syphilis, unless there are other signs of the disease. In most instances, they will perform a more expensive but accurate test that rarely comes out positive unless syphilitic infection is present or has existed in the past.

A distressing feature of the blood test for syphilis is that it can remain positive indefinitely, even when the treatment has cured the infection. This usually happens only if therapy with penicillin was delayed until the disease had become well established. In this situation, the persistently positive blood test is only an indication of a past infection. It is *not* a warning that further treatment is required, as long as adequate amounts of penicillin have already been administered.

Acquired Immune Deficiency Syndrome (AIDS)

The AIDS virus attacks and destroys the immune cells that normally protect us from infections. The skin, more than any other organ, reflects the symptoms of this lethal disease; skin infections of all kinds occur frequently in patients afflicted with AIDS. Viral infections such as warts, molluscum contagiosum, herpes simplex, herpes zoster, and chicken pox often evolve into unusually severe forms in AIDS patients. Similarly, fungus infections such as candidiasis and ringworm are intractable in AIDS victims and respond poorly to treatment with medications that are normally quite effective.

A tumor of blood-vessel cells called Kaposi's sarcoma is often one of the early manifestations of AIDS. It appears as purplish lines, spots, or swellings on the skin surface or inside the mouth and sometimes throughout the intestinal tract. An unrelated form of Kaposi's sarcoma has long been recognized among elderly Italian and Jewish men. This old man's form of the disease is usually compatible with a long life.

Seborrheic dermatitis (see chapter 2) occurs in AIDS patients in a far more extensive and severe form than it does in people with a healthy immune system. (In some patients with AIDS, the dermatitis improves with treatment with an antifungal antibiotic, suggesting that this common rash may be caused by an unidentified fungus.) In addition to seborrheic dermatitis, AIDS patients suffer from various forms of eczema and dry skin rashes. With the myriad of skin findings, it is not surprising that the dermatologist is often the first physician to consider and confirm the diagnosis of AIDS.

10 BITES AND STINGS

There are insects that bite a person and then crawl or fly away, and other insects that bite and then take up residence on the skin. The latter condition, where the insect finds the environment of the skin suitable for living and reproduction, is called an *infestation*. The distinction between bites and infestations is more than academic. Simple bites can be treated by local application of soothing lotions (and avoiding the insect in question). In the case of infestations, elimination of the infesting insects is the only treatment, and that may require treating the skin with chemicals that are lethal to the infesting creatures but may be irritating or toxic to the human host as well.

Patients are often chagrined when they are told that an undiagnosed rash is nothing more than a collection of insect bites; their response to this diagnosis may range from denial to disgust and embarrassment. These reactions, although understandable, are unreasonable. With few exceptions, neglect or poor personal hygiene have little to do with acquiring bites or infestations. In most cultures in the world, coexisting with insects and other biting creatures is viewed as an insignificant experience of daily life.

Let's take a look at the insects that cause most of the annoyance.

Fleas

In most households in the United States, the ordinary flea is the frequent cause of multiple insect bites. Fleas are content (and actually prefer) to live on domestic pets, but if the pet is de-flea'ed or relegated to a cold, out-of-doors environment, the fleas will happily settle for a human-blood diet.

Fleas are tiny wingless creatures possessing extraordinarily powerful legs that enable them to jump several feet in the air. Thus most flea bites in humans occur on the ankles and legs, unless the flea-ridden pet sleeps on the bed with its owner and the bites occur during the night.

Like most insect bites, flea bites appear in clusters or in a linear arrangement, since the lazy flea doesn't like to travel very far for his second and third meal. Flea bites appear as small, hivelike swellings with a central blood spot where the flea's mouth has penetrated the skin. Since the skin reaction is primarily an allergic response, and not everyone is allergic to the flea's saliva, bites may range from barely perceptible papules to large, impressive blisters. This variation in response explains why all persons living in a flea-infested environment do not necessarily show signs of being bitten.

The elimination of fleas from the home is not a simple matter. There are sprays and aerosol bombs available in pet stores and through veterinarians, but fleas and flea eggs, hidden away in furniture and deep-piled carpets, are often impervious to the assaults of amateur exterminators. Fortunately, the onset of cold weather may solve a summer flea problem when other methods fail.

Obviously, the source of the fleas must also be treated by a veterinarian at the same time the home is being de-flea'ed. If not, the pet will reinfect the home or vice versa.

For severe cases, there are insect repellents that will deter flea bites. The chemical diethylmetatoluamide (deet) is the most effective active ingredient. Insect repellents should be sprayed on the feet and lower legs or other sites prone to flea bites until the flea problem in the home has been resolved. But do treat insect repellents with respect—these chemicals are powerful and potentially harmful, especially to small children. Use them only when necessary and then sparingly.

135

Spiders

Most spiders are industrious creatures that improve the environment by capturing and devouring small insects. The typical attic and cellar spider does not bite human beings. There are a few spider species, however, that do not like to be trifled with.

Anyone who has read a few mystery novels is familiar with the infamous *black widow spider,* so called because the female of the species kills her mate after copulation. This coal-black creature measures only half an inch in length and can be identified by a distinctive red hourglass-shaped marking on the midportion of its body.

Although the black widow bite produces only mild local discomfort, the venom may spread throughout the body and cause an acute illness characterized by abdominal pain and vomiting, severe muscle aches, and neurological symptoms. If the spider bite is recognized as the origin of the illness, then it can be treated with a commercial serum that inactivates the poison venom. The black widow bite is not as serious as some of the fictional sources imply, but the mortality rate without treatment does approach 10 percent.

The *brown recluse spider* is a more common cause of a serious spider bite. This shy creature hides out in barns, garages, and basements and attacks only when disturbed. Like the black widow, the brown recluse can be identified by its distinctive markings—a dark brown violin-shaped design that covers its head and torso. Like the black widow the bite may be virtually painless, but within hours a blister or pustule develops at the site of the venom injection. In more severe reactions, the toxic chemical spreads beyond the bite area and causes a gangrenous ulceration of the skin, sometimes accompanied by fever, chills, headache, and muscle pains.

Appropriate first-aid measures for a brown recluse spider bite are directed at limiting the spread of the toxic venom. Apply cold applications to the bite site, keep the person still, and, if possible, elevate the portion of the body that sustained the bite. See a doctor as soon as possible. Although there is no specific remedy for brown recluse spider bites, a physician may excise the bite area and administer antibiotics and corticosteroids, which may prevent later infection and sloughing of the skin.

Ticks

Ticks are eight-legged creatures that are found in wooded areas in all parts of the United States. Their major importance lies in the fact that they transmit the organisms (spirochetes) that cause several serious infectious diseases, including Rocky Mountain spotted fever and Lyme disease (see chapter 9).

Mosquitoes, Flies, and Gnats

One of the great mysteries of outdoor life is the attraction that some people seem to present for these fly-and-bite creatures. Studies suggest that subtle differences in body odor, skin temperature, and the amount and composition of sweat either attract or repel these insects.

Some physicians and entomologists believe thiamine (vitamin B_1) may help. When excreted in the sweat, thiamine produces an odor that is said to repel mosquitoes and other winged insects. This has not been confirmed. The most conventional time-tested form of protection can be purchased in the form of a commercial insect repellent that contains diethylmetatoluamide (deet), dimethyl phthalate, or ethylhexanediol. Again, use these chemicals with caution, especially on small children.

Bees

It has been estimated that in the United States more people die annually from bee stings than from poison snake bites. A fatal bee sting reaction occurs only if a previous sting has induced a state of allergy in the person, which means that circulating antibodies to the bee venom are present and are ready to react with it.

More often, bee stings cause a nonallergic reaction, characterized by redness and swelling at the sting site. In the absence of allergy, even multiple stings are not dangerous or life-threatening.

Among the common bees in the United States, it is the honey-bee—unlike the wasp, hornet, or yellowjacket—that may leave a stinger in the skin. Before applying any medication to the sting, try to remove the honeybee stinger by gently scraping the skin with a knife or fingernail. (Vigorous efforts to remove the stinger serve only to release more venom into the sting wound.) Once the stinger is out, an application of ice or cold water, mud packs or meat tenderizer, or anesthetic creams and lotions will decrease the pain and swelling. Apply some anti-bacterial ointment to prevent infection. Often an antihistamine is prescribed, which rarely reduces the pain and swelling, although it can help to relieve any allergic reactions.

Allergic Reactions and Treatment Although it takes 500 or more simultaneous bee stings to introduce enough bee venom to kill an average-sized man, one sting can be fatal to the highly allergic person. This lethal form of allergic reaction is called *anaphylaxis* or *anaphylactic shock.* Within seconds after the sting, the bee venom reacts with antibodies in the bloodstream that trigger the release of large amounts of histamine from the cells throughout the body. It is largely histamine that causes the symptoms of anaphylaxis: swelling of the skin and hives, cold sweats and pallor, and a sharp drop in blood pressure. If not treated immediately, the anaphylactic victim may lapse into un-consciousness and die.

Epinephrine is the single most important medication for the emergency treatment of anaphylactic shock. If injected under the skin or, when possible, directly into a vein, it will act quickly to raise blood pressure and open up the constricted breathing passages. Antihistamines and corticosteroids are slower to act and are given to counteract the allergic reaction only after ep-inephrine has reversed the shock.

Fortunately, allergy to bee sting venom is not always mani-fested by a life-threatening anaphylaxis. But any allergic re-actions such as hives, joint swelling, or even prolonged swelling at the sting site imply that a more serious, possibly life-threat-ening reaction might occur with subsequent stings. Individuals who have experienced even the most mild allergic reaction to a bee sting are well advised to carry an emergency kit with them routinely in case they experience another sting. Most of the kits contain a preloaded syringe of Adrenalin, antihistamine pills, tourniquets, and instructions on how to handle such an allergic emergency.

Allergists are most qualified to investigate the possibility of bee sting allergy. If an allergic state exists, as determined by skin and blood tests, then desensitization with injections of bee venom extract may decrease the chances of a serious allergic reaction should another sting occur. But since this type of desensitization is imperfect, it stands to reason that highly allergic individuals should avoid environments that are attractive to bees. Heavily flowered areas and summer picnics with abundant bee-attracting foods should be off limits. Similarly, allergic individuals should avoid using perfume or after-shave lotions and wearing bright-colored clothing in the summer months.

Lice

Among the creatures that live on the human skin, two stand out above all others because of their universality and their persistence throughout history. They are the louse and the scabies mite. Fortunately, the human race has not been subject to fatal epidemics of louse-transmitted typhus in the past fifty years, but nuisance infections caused by this six-legged creature are widespread.

The sexually transmitted infection of the crab louse *Pediculus hominus pubis* is discussed in chapter 9. *Pediculus hominus capitis,* a cousin of the crab louse, prefers to lay its eggs on the scalp hairs. Like the crab louse, the head louse is sometimes ignored, or misdiagnosed by the afflicted person or, if the patient is a child, by the parents. Numerous bottles of medicated shampoos are often purchased in an attempt to eliminate an "itchy scalp" or "dandruff." On close inspection by a physician, however, the "dandruff flakes" prove to be louse eggs (nits) that are firmly attached to the hairs and, unlike dandruff scales, not easily brushed off.

Treatment Once recognized, head lice are not difficult to eradicate. A physician can prescribe a shampoo containing lindane (gamma benzene hexachloride), which kills lice and their un-born offspring on contact. One application will usually do the job; once treatment is completed, the remaining nits that are still firmly attached to the hair shaft can be removed by fine-combing the hair with a solution of one part water and one part plain vinegar. There are some over-the-counter shampoos for lice, but they are not as effective as shampoos containing lin-dane. Lindane is safe to use, even for children, as long as in-structions on the bottle are carefully followed.

Body Lice Infections caused by *Pediculus hominus corporis,* the body louse, are usually associated with poverty and poor hy-giene. Body lice epidemics can occur also in wartime or follow-ing some natural catastrophe that disrupts normal sanitation. The body louse feeds off the skin but spends most of the time hidden away in the nooks and crannies of clothing. A long-standing infestation by body lice presents a picture of a widespread, scratched-up rash, discoloration of the skin, and running sores from bacterial infection, a consequence of con-stant scratching. While treatment with lindane is in order, equal attention should be paid to the circumstances that made the environment suitable for this kind of infestation.

Scabies

Although the great scabies epidemic of the past two decades appears to be tapering off, the disease is still very much around. Scabies, a highly contagious skin disease, is an intensely itchy rash caused by *Sarcoptes scabiei,* a tiny mite that cannot be seen with the naked eye. The reasons for the epidemic of this disease are not clear. Some scientists attribute it to changes in social and sexual mores that tend to encourage the spread of body contact disease. Another theory relates the epidemic to a world-wide reduction in immunity to the mite. This latter theory sug-gests that the recurrent scabies epidemics are inevitable cyclic phenomena. Although once believed to be a disease of lower socioeconomic groups, scabies affects people of all ages, races, and classes.

The scabies rash appears weeks or even months after inti-

140

mate or persistent indirect contact with an infested person. Gradually, itchy bumps appear on the sides of the fingers, arms, chest, and genital area. Eventually, the entire body, except the head and face, may be covered with the rash. Among the scratches and irritations it is usually possible to identify several linear sores, called *burrows,* where the scabies mite is marching along under the skin depositing eggs that will one day hatch to become young mites.

Diagnosis and Treatment The present epidemic has spawned some strange-looking rashes that are quite different from this typical pattern. When in doubt, a physician who suspects scabies can attempt to prove the diagnosis by scraping the skin off a burrow and examining the material under a microscope. This technique may reveal the mite, or signs that the mite has been there—namely, the eggs or feces it has left behind. Since scraping examinations are often negative even in the face of active infection, many physicians will treat scabies based upon a clinical diagnosis.

Scabies is most often treated with lindane (gamma benzene hexachloride), the same medication that is used to treat lice infestations. Lindane lotion is applied over the entire body, from the neck down. After twelve to twenty-four hours the medication is removed by a bath or shower. Although one application is sufficient to kill all the adult mites, some physicians recommend a second application, one to seven days later, to kill any mites that may have hatched after the treatment.

Patients often decide to retreat themselves because of persistent itching that may continue for weeks, even after all the mites are dead. This can be a dangerous practice because lindane is a toxic chemical that can be injurious to the nervous system if excessive amounts are absorbed into the body. For this reason, some physicians prefer to treat scabies with other medications, particularly if infants or very young children are infested. A chemical called *crotamiton,* and 5 percent sulfur ointment, are alternative topical medications that are used to kill the scabies mite.

Patients with postscabies syndrome, the persistent itch and rash experienced long after the mites have been killed with

141

appropriate therapy, should use anti-itch lotions, antihistamines, and sometimes a course of oral corticosteroids prescribed by the dermatologist. Such stubborn symptoms are not surprising, however, since much of the scabies rash is an allergic reaction to the presence of mites on the skin.

Jellyfish

Ocean bathers can suffer painful stings from contact with some species of jellyfish, particularly the Portuguese man-of-war and sea anemones that carry poisonous stingers on their tentacles. Painful hivelike welts appear, often in a line where the tentacles have touched the skin. If sufficient venom is absorbed into the body, then other symptoms can follow, including headache, dizziness, and muscle cramps. Serious shocklike allergic reactions are, fortunately, rare.

Treatment Immediate treatment on the beach is possible, if certain items are available. The painful sting can be relieved by applying a weak acid, such as vinegar, to the welts. The pain can also be alleviated with cold applications (damp sand will do) or with meat tenderizer.

Delayed reactions may occur days after the sting, in the form of hives, pigmented rashes, or firm bumps that can take weeks or months to resolve. If such reactions occur, see a dermatologist for further treatment.

11 THE SUN AND SKIN CANCER

According to contemporary theory, the various rays emanating from the sun carry energy and travel on waves in an up-and-down roller-coaster pattern. The different rays of the sun are characterized by *wavelength,* or the measurement between the peaks of two successive waves. The shortest rays, the gamma and X rays, are found at one end of the solar spectrum; the very long micro and radio waves are at the other end. The rays that most affect the skin, the ultraviolet and light rays, fall between these two extremes.

Radiation as it leaves the surface of the sun is very different from the sun rays that strike the earth. Fortunately for all living creatures, the gamma and X rays, as well as some of the very short ultraviolet waves, are absorbed by gases in the ozone layer of the earth's atmosphere. According to recent scientific research, however, damage to the ozone layer caused by halogenated hydrocarbons found in aerosol sprays and other man-made gas pollutants now permits more short, ultraviolet waves to reach the earth's surface. This development is likely to translate into an increase of skin cancers in the years ahead.

More than half the sun's rays that penetrate the atmosphere and reach the earth's surface are ultraviolet and visible light rays. These rays are measured on a very small scale, that of nanometers (one nanometer is equal to .000001 meter). The ultraviolet light that reaches the earth measures between 290 and 400 nanometers; the visible light is in the 400-to-700-nanometer range. In studying the effects of ultraviolet light on the skin and other biological systems, scientists have subdivided ultraviolet rays even further. The shorter, higher-energy rays that produce sunburn are called *UVB,* and measure from 290 to 320 nanometers. The longer, low-energy waves that measure 320 to 400 nanometers are called *UVA.* These waves don't burn, but they are important factors in tanning as well as in many forms of sun allergy.

Sunburn

Many of us can recall when a brisk, skin-peeling sunburn was considered the red badge of courage, a painful memory of a day at the beach or fishing on the lake. A new, sun-wary generation is better informed; today, for the most part, severe sunburns are accidental and not by design.

Sunburn depends upon several factors, including the number of hours of exposure as well as the time of day you select for sunning. At midday, when the sun is directly overhead, the sun's rays travel a short, direct course to the earth's surface and strike the skin after a minimal amount of filtering by the atmosphere. In contrast, when the sun is low in the sky in the late afternoon, the rays travel a longer, more oblique path through the atmosphere and are maximally filtered.

The inevitability of sunburn will also depend on the amount of sun exposure you have previously received. If your skin has had a chance to mobilize its defenses with sun-stimulated thickening of the epidermis and skin-pigment formation, then you may avoid a sunburn.

In this regard, skin type cannot be ignored, and we usually speak of six general types: *Types 1* and *2* will burn easily and tan minimally, if at all. These are the very fair-skinned individuals with blond or red hair. *Types 5* and *6* are heavily pigmented individuals who tan easily and seldom experience any sunburn. Most of the Caucasian population fall in the in-between categories of *types 3* and *4*; they burn sometimes but gradually develop a protective tan.

Symptoms of sunburn appear two to four hours after sun exposure. The first sign is redness of the skin, which is soon followed by swelling, pain, and sensitivity to touch—sunburn victims are extremely uncomfortable when anything, including their own clothing, touches the skin. The sunburn reaction reaches a peak after twenty-four hours and continues for another day or two, at which time the skin cells begin to scale off and the postsunburn peel becomes apparent. During the first twenty-four hours radiation from heat in the reddened skin is so intense that the body reacts with chills and fever. (Chills are often due to the effects of a cold shower, which at the time may seem like a logical treatment for burning skin, but definitely is not.)

Treatment Sunburn, like so many common medical problems, is not easy to treat. There are no specific medications that will effectively "cure" a sunburn, for the simple reason that the chemical mechanisms that underlie the reaction are not completely understood.

Proper first-aid treatment for sunburn generally includes the use of tepid baths or showers, soothing creams or lotions, and aspirin taken orally. Tepid baths are recommended to avoid chills. The addition of baking soda, bath oil, or an oatmeal powder to the bath water increases the soothing effect. Creams or lotions that contain very small quantities of menthol or phenol provide some pain relief, and are safer than the over-the-counter lotions that contain "-caine" anesthetics, which sometimes cause allergic reactions. If your sunburn is on the mild side, a soothing over-the-counter corticosteroid cream or a bland ointment with aloe vera as its main ingredient will reduce the unpleasant itch-burn sensation.

Aspirin is one of the safest and most useful medications for the systemic treatment of sunburn—it has anti-inflammatory properties as well as the more familiar pain-relieving qualities. Many sunburn patients do not appreciate this fact, and choose to ignore their doctor's advice to take ten grains (two tablets) of aspirin every four hours for a two- to three-day period. Ibuprofen or one of the other nonsteroidal anti-inflammatory drugs may be almost as effective, and can be used in place of aspirin. With very severe sunburns, in order to reduce the pain, redness, and swelling to more tolerable levels, it is safe to take small doses of systemic corticosteroids for a few days—with a doctor's prescription.

Tanning

Tanning results from exposure to UVB, the sunburn rays. UVA, the long, ultraviolet waves, also contribute to the tanning process. This fact gives credence to the advertising claim of some sunscreens and tanning lotions that claim to block out UVB, urging customers to "tan without burning." Unfortunately, tanning as well as burning can lead to premature aging of the skin and to skin cancer.

Tanning takes place in two distinct phases. Immediately upon exposure to ultraviolet light, the melanin already present in the epidermal cells is oxidized from a brown to a darker brown color. At the same time, the melanin granules are redistributed in the epidermal cells in a manner that creates further darkening of the skin. This stage of tanning, however, is a transient one, and darkening disappears very rapidly when the light stimulation is removed.

A more permanent tan begins to appear two to three days after exposure to the burning rays and, to a lesser extent, after exposure to the long-wave, ultraviolet light. In this delayed tanning process, the melanocytes are activated to produce new melanin and to transfer it to the surrounding epidermal cells. Since the long-wave UVA can initiate delayed tanning, it is possible to screen out the sunburn rays and still acquire a tan, but this will require more intensive sun exposure.

Although suntan is considered to be attractive, and society places a positive social and economic value on tanned skin, most of us would be better off without it. A suntan indicates that the skin is receiving large amounts of radiation and has been forced to use the tanning mechanism to protect itself from further radiation damage.

CUMULATIVE DAMAGE TO THE SKIN

The adverse effects of solar radiation are cumulative. Significant sun damage does not appear on the skin after one or two episodes of sunburn, but after years of regular and prolonged sun exposure. For those living in warm, sunny climates, where year-round, outdoor living is frequently an economic necessity, as in the case of farmers and ranchers, severely sun-damaged skin is not uncommon by the age of forty or fifty. In more temperate climates, similar skin changes are seen less frequently and in older people.

The degenerative skin changes associated with sun exposure appear on the areas of maximal exposure: the face, the hands, the V area of the upper chest, and the back of the neck. The skin in these areas becomes wrinkled, thinned out, dry, and irregularly discolored. In some areas, such as the back of the neck, the skin assumes a leathery consistency with deep criss-crossing furrows. Severely sun-damaged skin forms the terrain out of which sprout a variety of benign and malignant skin growths. Prevention of these complications begins with the use of an effective sunscreen.

Sunscreens

Since outdoor living has become a part of our life-style and is not likely to change, moderate to excessive sun exposure is largely inevitable for most of us. Sun protection, then, should become a part of our routine through the regular application of a protective sunscreen.

Sunscreens are preparations that you apply to your skin to prevent the damaging ultraviolet waves from entering the epidermal cells and penetrating to the deeper levels of the skin. There are two general types of sunscreens available. Ordinary zinc oxide ointment is an example of a screen that blocks ultraviolet and light rays because of the physical nature of the zinc oxide particles. This type of opaque screen forms an impenetrable barrier to all of the burning and tanning rays, and is most useful in protecting limited areas of the skin from prolonged sun exposure. There are a few commercial preparations containing zinc oxide or titanium dioxide that are available for complete screening. These heavy, opaque preparations are not easily applied and are not cosmetically acceptable to most consumers.

The most popular sunscreens filter out limited portions of

147

the ultraviolet spectrum through the absorption properties of specific chemicals. The most widely used formulations contain para-aminobenzoic acid (PABA), or a PABA derivative in an alcohol, gel, or lubricating lotion. To date, PABA is the most effective chemical screen for UVB and, if used properly, will significantly reduce your chance of sunburn.

Sometimes irritant or allergic dermatitis occurring from the use of PABA preparations may prevent you from using this particular sunscreen. A preexisting allergy to a black dye (para-phenylenediamine), anesthetics of the "-caine" group, or sulfa drugs may also result in a cross-sensitivity to the chemically similar PABA preparations.

Another large group of commercial sunscreens contains benzophenones and/or cinnamates, two broad-spectrum screens that absorb both UVB and UVA waves. These chemicals are suitable substitutes if you experience irritation or allergic reactions from the PABA preparations. The broad-spectrum screens not only provide you maximum protection but sometimes are useful in sun allergy or skin diseases that are made worse by exposure to UVA waves.

Several well-known cosmetic suntan lotions contain a chemical called *homomenthyl salicylate*. This ingredient makes for a rather ineffectual screen that you should not rely on for either partial or complete sunburn protection.

Sun Protection Factor Most of the commercial sunscreens have been assigned a rating to denote their relative protective value against the sun's rays. This "sun protection factor," or SPF, is a measurement of the exposure time required to turn the skin red with the sunscreen in place. A sunscreen with an SPF of 15, for example, will permit fifteen times as much exposure as normally tolerated. In the past few years the pharmaceutical and cosmetic industries have engaged in an SPF competition, pushing the numbers up beyond fifteen. Today, sunscreens with SPFs of 30, 40, and even 50 are available. What are you to make of all of this? Most photobiologists feel that a sunscreen with an SPF in the 15-to-20 range provides you with sufficient protection in all circumstances. Sunscreens with higher SPFs are not harmful, but neither are they more effective.

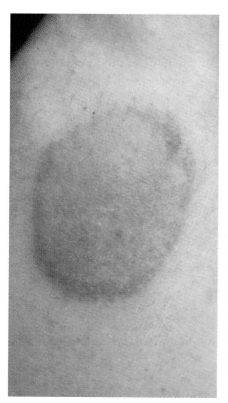 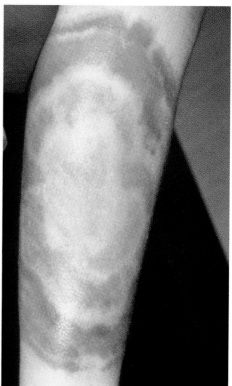

Left: A skin rash—the earliest sign
of Lyme disease. This typical rash,
about two inches in diameter, was
caused by a bite on the leg. Rashes
may also have a central clear area.
Treatment at this stage can prevent
later complications.

Right: Another variety of rash,
consisting of concentric red bands.
This one is on the calf. Rashes
commonly form within a few weeks of
the tick bite. They usually don't itch
but often are warm to the touch.

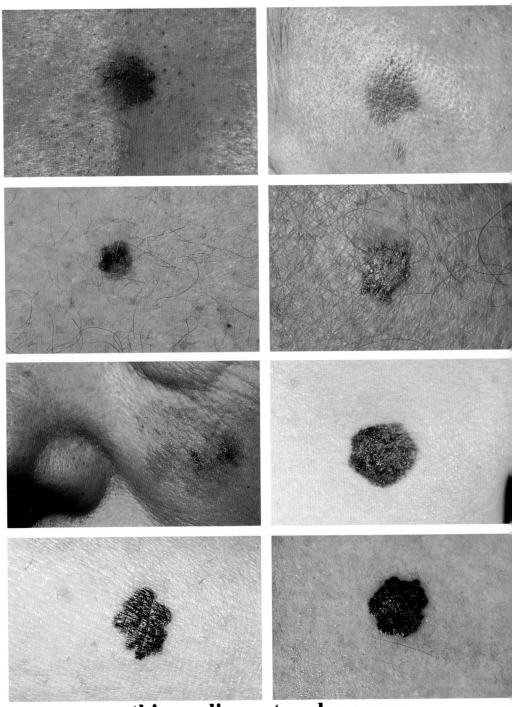

thin malignant melanomas
—excellent prognosis

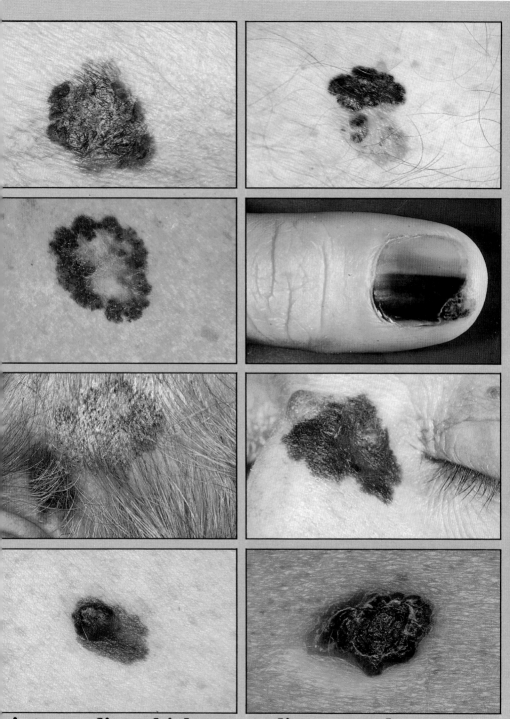

intermediate thickness malignant melanomas
—less predictable prognosis

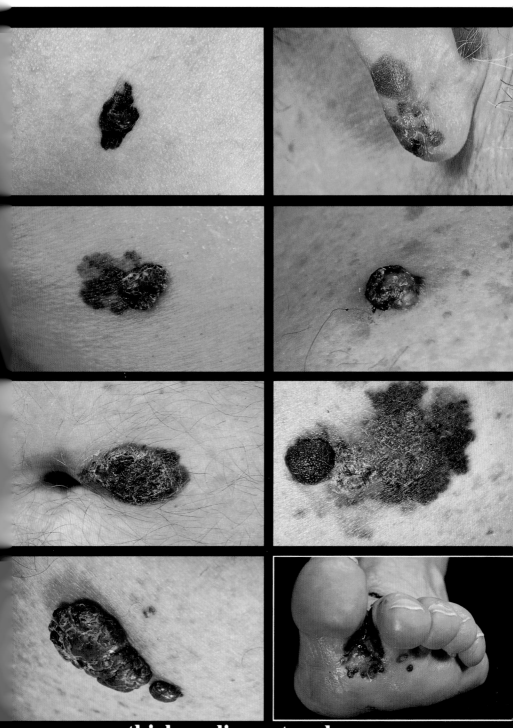

thick malignant melanomas
—poor prognosis

It is reassuring to know that the SPF value claimed by the manufacturers of sunscreens *is* accurate. In a June 1988 *Consumer Reports* evaluation of sunscreens, not only were the SPF values confirmed, but the "waterproof" claim (i.e., maintaining the SPF stated on the label after four twenty-minute swims) was also validated (see Ratings charts in the appendix). Nevertheless, none of the sunscreens is completely waterproof, and it makes good sense to reapply a sunscreen several times during the course of a day of outdoor activity.

Despite the cosmetic industry's progress, the perfect sunscreen has yet to be formulated, and you should avoid indiscriminate sunbathing. Wide-brimmed hats and umbrellas can offer additional protection, but not from ultraviolet light that is reflected off water, sandy beaches, and even city pavements. There are times when the best "screen" may be a room with drawn shades.

Tretinoin

Most of what we perceive as aging skin is actually damage caused by the external environment, mainly from the sun. No known drug can halt the progression of intrinsic aging. But it appears that sun-induced aging can be partially reversed by *retinoic acid,* a vitamin-A compound also known as *tretinoin,* which is the active ingredient in Retin-A. A recent medical study reported that the drug (long a mainstay of acne treatment; see page 46) was applied daily for sixteen weeks on the skin of thirty volunteers, ages fifty to seventy. It decreased fine lines (but did not alter deep character lines), lightened brown spots, and gave the skin a healthy, rosy appearance.

Short-term side effects of Retin-A were common. Nearly all patients in the study experienced skin inflammation for periods of two weeks to several months. More than a third had to be treated with a steroid cream, and three patients quit the study because of the severity of skin irritation. For most patients, irritation subsided after a time as the skin developed a tolerance to the drug.

Above all, anyone who uses Retin-A should use a sunscreen when outdoors. Using it without a sunscreen is not only irritating to the skin but may actually accelerate premature aging and increase the risk of skin cancer.

Pregnant women should not use the product until there is firm assurance that it is safe; the drug is chemically related to the oral acne drug Accutane, which has caused birth defects.

The Food and Drug Administration has not yet approved tretinoin as an anti-photoaging medication, although some dermatologists are already prescribing it to their patients. (No federal law prevents physicians from prescribing any approved drug for whatever use they deem appropriate.) It will take additional studies involving a large number of subjects using tretinoin for months, probably years, to gain more information about the persistence of favorable changes and the side effects of long-term usage. Since its benefits are cosmetic rather than health-related, the FDA must make sure that the risks are negligible before granting approval.

CANCER OF THE SKIN

Chronic sun exposure or sunburn is the major causal factor in the development of skin cancer. The areas of the body that receive maximum sun exposure are also the areas where the great majority of skin cancers proliferate: the head and neck, the upper torso, and, in women, the lower extremities.

The three common forms of skin cancer are: basal cell carcinoma, squamous cell carcinoma, and malignant melanoma.

Basal Cell Carcinoma

Basal cell carcinoma is by far the most common form of skin malignancy. In the United States it outranks the runner-up, squamous cell carcinoma, by at least a ten-to-one margin. Basal cell tumors are a relatively benign form of cancer, and almost never spread from their site of origin. They are capable of growing deep into the skin and underlying tissue, but the cancer cells do not enter the bloodstream or lymph channels or spread to distant parts of the body. This is not to suggest that these skin growths should be ignored. Their ability to invade and destroy skin and adjacent tissue can lead to ulcerations, infections, and serious cosmetic deformities.

Basal cell cancers are directly related to sun exposure. They develop most often (as do other types of skin cancer) in people with fair skin, freckles, blue, green, or gray eyes, and blond hair, and who tan poorly because of inadequate amounts of protective melanin pigment. These cancers occur rarely in black people and infrequently in Hispanics or dark-skinned Caucasians. In the United States, the incidence of basal cell carcinoma is considerably higher in the South and Southwest than in the North.

It's also true that radiation other than the ultraviolet rays of the sun can predispose a person to the development of a basal cell carcinoma. Years after X-ray therapy was administered for their severe acne conditions, patients so treated developed basal cell cancers on the treated areas of the face. Arsenic, once used to treat asthma and anemia, has also been known to cause the growth of multiple basal cell cancers some twenty years or more after ingestion of the cell-poisoning "medication."

Diagnosis Basal cell cancers come in many different shapes, sizes, and even colors. They are not always easily identifiable to the trained eye, much less to the layperson.

If there is such a thing as a typical basal cell skin cancer, it might be described as a pinkish, smooth-surfaced, solid, slowly growing papule that bleeds easily from relatively minor trauma. Other less typical forms of basal cell carcinoma appear as flat red spots, pigmented growths, skin ulcers that fail to heal by themselves, and white, fibrous areas that could be mistaken for scar tissue. The variation is so great and the atypical so common that self-diagnosis is not only foolhardy but impossible. The physician who examines such a skin growth must rely on a biopsy and microscopic study to confirm or refute a suspicion that a growth is cancer.

Treatment There are many methods of treating basal cell cancers, including surgery, chemotherapy, and radiation. Surgical treatment might take the form of an excision of the tumor followed by suturing the wound together or placing a skin graft, if the wound is too large to close with sutures. This type of surgery might be performed by a dermatologist, a plastic surgeon, or a general surgeon. By and large it is dermatologists who remove most basal cell cancers by a surgical technique called *electrodesiccation and curettage*. This method employs a rounded cutting instrument, the curette, and electrocautery to destroy the tumor. A relatively new surgical technique, *Mohs surgery*, examines the excised tumor as soon as it is removed to ensure that the margins are clear and that no cancer cells have been left behind. This technique is particularly useful for basal cell cancers that have recurred after some other form of treatment, and for growths where it is difficult to see where the tumor ends and healthy tissue begins. Another method is *cryosurgery*, a process that destroys and removes the tumor by freezing it, usually with super-cold liquid nitrogen.

Superficial basal cell cancers can be effectively treated with topical 5-fluorouracil, a method of treatment best described as chemotherapy. Radiotherapy offers another nonsurgical alternative. It is often selected for elderly people or those who are unable to tolerate a surgical procedure.

The striking fact about all of the methods employed to treat basal cell cancers is that the cure rate is much the same for all—over 90 percent for most surgical techniques and radiation—as long as the doctor using the technique is skilled in its application. Basal cell carcinomas that recur after treatment (usually within a few years) are generally treated by another modality, frequently Mohs microscopically controlled surgery.

Squamous Cell Carcinoma

Squamous cell carcinomas are as varied in appearance as basal cell carcinomas. The often-described sore that won't heal or a crusted, heaped-up nodule are different but accurate descriptions of squamous cell carcinoma. Like basal cell carcinomas, squamous cell cancers grow on sun-damaged skin, frequently arising from red, often tender scaly spots called *solar keratoses*. These precancerous lesions are very common in the elderly and in fair-skinned individuals. Fortunately, the likelihood of a solar keratosis developing into cancer is rather small. *Bowen's disease* is a squamous cell carcinoma that is only on the skin surface and confined to the epidermis.

Squamous cell cancer often arises in scar tissue, at sites of previous burns, and on skin that has undergone radiation damage. Squamous cell cancers that grow on the lip or inside the mouth are more invasive than those that arise on the skin surface from solar keratoses.

Treatment Most squamous cell carcinomas are removed surgically. X-ray therapy is reserved for special situations where surgery would be too involved or deforming, such as on the eyelids, tip of nose, or lips.

Malignant Melanoma

Malignant melanoma was once a rare form of skin cancer, but its incidence has increased tenfold in the past fifty years. Among Caucasians in the United States, the lifetime risk has risen to close to one in a hundred. No one is certain why melanoma has increased to near-epidemic proportions, but the evidence favors a change in our habits of sun exposure that dates back some thirty to forty years.

Melanoma is the most lethal of the three forms of skin cancer and it claimed close to 6,000 lives in the United States in 1988. The death rate from melanoma is increasing at a rate faster than any other cancer, with the exception of lung cancer in women.

The earlier melanoma is diagnosed and treated, the better the prognosis. In Australia, where a fair-skinned population experiences much sun exposure, the incidence of melanoma is very high. In Queensland a public educational program has decreased the death rate from melanoma despite an increasing number of new cases. Early diagnosis and treatment have paid off.

Melanomas are pigment cell cancers. At one time it was thought that all melanomas were once pigmented moles that had undergone a malignant change. It is now recognized that most melanomas develop on perfectly normal skin. Only 25 percent or less develop from a preexisting mole that may have been present for years. It is obvious, therefore, that new, pigmented growths in adults can be early melanomas.

What to Look For The following "ABC" characteristics of pigmented skin growths should arouse the suspicion of both doctor and layperson:

- "A" stands for *asymmetry*. If a line is drawn down the middle of a melanoma, one half will be different in shape and contour from the other half. This is not the case with benign moles, which tend to be rounded and symmetrical.
- "B" stands for *border*. The borders of melanomas are apt to be scalloped or indistinct. They have a blurred margin that fades into the surrounding skin.
- "C" stands for *color*. Unlike the homogeneous brown color of most moles, melanoma coloring is variegated—there are shades of tan, brown, black, red, blue, and white.

So the key to melanoma diagnosis is irregularity: irregular shape, irregular borders, irregular coloration. In addition to the ABCs, other warning signs in preexisting moles are:

1. Change in size—especially sudden or continuous enlargement.

2. Change in elevation—especially the raising of a part of a pigmented area that used to be flat or only slightly elevated.

3. Change in surface—especially scaliness, erosion, oozing, crusting, ulceration, or bleeding.

4. Change in surrounding skin—especially redness, swelling, or the development of colored blemishes next to, but not part of, the pigmented area.

5. Change in sensation—especially itchiness, tenderness, or pain.

6. Change in consistency—especially softening or hardening.

Diagnosis and treatment Melanomas can grow on the surface of the skin for months or even years. At some point they may go into a vertical growth phase and extend down into the deeper portions of the skin, where the malignant cells can enter the lymph channels and blood vessels, and be carried throughout the body. When this happens, the melanoma obviously becomes thicker. Calculating the thickness of melanoma determines its curability. Melanomas that are less than 1/32 inch thick have close to a 100 percent cure rate. Melanomas that are thicker have a proportionately poorer prognosis.

The diagnosis of melanoma is established after your dermatologist obtains a tissue sample (biopsy) from the pigmented lesion in question. A skilled pathologist will be able to recognize the cancer cells and other microscopic features that will confirm the diagnosis. The melanoma is then removed surgically with a wide and deep margin of surrounding normal tissue in order to remove any malignant cells that may have strayed from the main growth itself. Unfortunately, despite the best surgical efforts, melanoma has a high rate of mortality because of its tendency to spread to other parts of the body.

You should realize that the information provided here about melanoma and other skin growths is of limited value in terms of self-diagnosis. To overdescribe skin tumors and present "general concepts" may only lead you to a false sense of security. Different advice is needed in the form of that old adage: It's better to be safe than sorry. When a skin growth changes in character or in some other way arouses your suspicion, consult a dermatologist immediately.

12 MOLES AND OTHER BENIGN SKIN GROWTHS

It is impossible to describe the characteristics of most skin growths so that they are instantly identifiable to you. A trained dermatologist spends years learning the typical and atypical features of dozens of skin tumors, and even with extensive experience, a biopsy and microscopic examination of tissue are often the only ways to arrive at a valid diagnosis.

As we have said, you are strongly advised not to attempt your own diagnosis of skin growths. It is hoped that the information in this chapter will educate and enlighten, but it will not make you an instant diagnostician. When in doubt, see your dermatologist.

MOLES

The origin of the word *mole*, used to describe a pigmented skin growth, or *nevus*, is obscure. It is possibly akin to the German word *Mal*, which means "spot." Moles are made up of collections of melanocytes—the pigment-manufacturing cells—that are normally scattered widely throughout the skin. These are the cells that synthesize melanin, which provides skin color as well as protection from ultraviolet radiation.

Moles first start to appear in early childhood. Initially, they appear as flat, dark brown spots, but with the passage of time they become elevated, rounded, and often a lighter shade of brown or pink. Some well-established moles may have a cluster of hairs growing from their surface.

By young adulthood, the average white-skinned person will have at least fifteen to twenty moles scattered over his or her body. New moles develop throughout life, but after adolescence they appear increasingly less frequently. The black population appears to develop fewer pigmented moles than do whites. Adult blacks, however, may develop multiple, small pigmented growths on their face that may be unsightly. These growths are not true moles, but rather smaller pigmented *seborrheic keratoses* (see page 160) that can be removed electrosurgically by a dermatologist.

At times it can be difficult to differentiate a mole from a freckle or from another flat brown mark called a *lentigo* (plural: *lentigines*). Freckles are small, flat brown spots that first appear on sun-exposed areas in childhood. Their presence is determined by hereditary factors, almost always appearing in families with red or blond hair. In contrast, lentigines develop late in life. They are dark brown in color and appear all over the body, but particularly on the face and top of the hands. Although they have nothing to do with the function of the liver, they are often referred to as "liver" spots, presumably because of their color. If desired, liver spots can be removed through the use of cryosurgery, using a liquid nitrogen spray, electrosurgery, or acid peeling.

Moles may pose a problem for several reasons. An unusual-looking mole, or a mole that has changed its appearance, raises the question of a serious form of skin cancer called *malignant melanoma* (see chapter 11). More often, moles attract attention because they are located in awkward places on the body, are irritated by clothing or shaving, or are unsightly. It is perfectly reasonable to remove a mole for any of these reasons. There is no convincing evidence, however, that a mole that is repeatedly rubbed or abraded is more likely to undergo a malignant change than a mole that is not subject to such trauma. On the other hand, excising (cutting out) a mole does *not* encourage any mole cells that might remain behind to change into cancer.

This curious misconception may have originated when occasional moles that had already become cancerous were removed but not subjected to microscopic study for signs of cancer. In these cases, if the mole grew back and was obviously malignant, it was assumed that the previous operation had caused the cancerous change.

Removal of Moles Realistically, it is not possible or even reasonable to remove all the moles on the human body. It has been estimated that all the dermatologists in the world could be kept busy excising moles twenty-four hours a day for a lifetime without completing this chore. A few dermatologists still recommend the prophylactic removal of moles in certain areas of the body—those flat, dark moles that appear on the palms, soles, or genital areas. But it is debatable whether these moles are more likely to become cancerous than are moles on other parts of the skin.

Most moles are removed for cosmetic reasons. As long as the patient appreciates the likely consequences of the removal of any particular mole, the procedure is usually satisfactory for doctor and patient. Many patients who seek the removal of a mole believe that the skin will heal in such a way that there will be no scar or evidence that a growth was once present on the skin. This is unrealistic. It is virtually impossible to cut out a mole or other skin growth and not leave some trace of the surgical procedure in the form of a scar, depression, or discoloration of the skin. It is up to the operating physician and the patient to determine whether the prospective surgery will lead to a better cosmetic situation than simply leaving the mole in place.

Congenital Moles

Some pigmented moles are present on the skin at birth. These "congenital" growths are frequently larger than the average mole that appears in childhood or adult life, occasionally covering a limb or a large portion of the body. There is some evidence to suggest that congenital moles are more likely to develop into a malignant tumor (melanoma) than moles that are acquired in childhood or adult life. For this reason, many dermatologists recommend the surgical removal of congenital moles when identified. Sometimes size or location make surgery difficult and impractical. In these cases, a dermatologist should examine the mole at regular intervals for any signs of malignant change.

Dysplastic Nevus Syndrome

There is another group of moles associated with an unusually high incidence of melanoma. These moles are called *dysplastic nevi*. The tendency to develop dysplastic nevi can be a familial trait often associated with a family history of malignant melanoma. Dysplastic nevi can be distinguished from normal moles because their color is variegated with shades of brown, tan, and pink, and unlike normal moles, they are not well demarcated— they have an ill-defined border that fades into the surrounding skin. Individuals born with the syndrome may grow a hundred or more moles on their torso over a period of years, well into their adult life. Since surgical removal of all these moles is impractical, periodic examination by a well-trained eye is an absolute necessity, as melanomas may develop in these moles or on the patient's normal skin. Those moles that do show suspicious changes are generally excised and examined microscopically.

KERATOSES

Excessive sun exposure and the passage of time conspire to create, on the skin of most people, a variety of spots, growths, and other signs of aging. To a large degree, the environment and hereditary factors will determine whether these degenerative skin growths will begin to appear in midlife or much later on. Keratoses are the most common benign growths that first appear in adult life and increase in number with age. *Seborrheic keratoses* are less age- and sun-dependent than the senile, or solar, keratoses, which are related to sun exposure as well as aging.

Seborrheic Keratoses

Seborrheic keratoses are flat or slightly elevated, brown, rough-surfaced spots that can grow by the dozens on the chest, back, face, and arms. A few seborrheic keratoses are tolerable since they are benign and do not change into any form of skin cancer. But when they are numerous they can be an unsightly and uncomfortable nuisance.

Treatment Fortunately, it is not difficult to remove seborrheic keratoses since they are soft and not very adherent to the skin surface. Most dermatologists will scrape them off with a curette (a rounded cutting instrument) after first freezing the skin for short-term anesthesia. The bleeding from this procedure is minimal and healing occurs rapidly without any permanent scar formation.

Seborrheic keratoses can also be removed electrosurgically through a process called *electrodesiccation*, which destroys the lesion with electric current. The lesion is then scraped off by a method known as curettage.

Solar Keratoses

Solar keratoses, clearly sun-related, appear on a background of sun-damaged skin—on the face, on the top of the hands and arms, and on the scalp in bald men. Fair-skinned people who have been exposed to the outdoors for years continue to grow many solar keratoses long after prolonged periods of sun exposure have been discontinued.

Solar keratoses are flat or slightly raised, red, scaly spots that may cause a burning or stinging sensation, and may be sensitive to the touch. They are considered to be a premalignant skin growth that can change into a form of skin cancer, the squamous cell carcinoma. But, since solar keratoses are common and squamous cell carcinomas rather rare, statistically most solar keratoses will not become cancerous. Therefore it is not necessary to remove every solar keratosis.

Treatment Methods of removal include electrosurgery with curettage, freezing, and chemical treatments. Chemotherapy with locally applied 5-fluorouracil is a favorite dermatological method for treating large numbers of solar keratoses at one time. When applied daily, this chemical causes an inflammation in and around the keratosis that, after three to four weeks, makes the growth self-destruct. The three-week period of treatment is not very pleasant, but if the discomfort and temporary unsightliness can be tolerated, the end results are usually quite good.

Removing solar keratoses is much like pulling weeds out of the garden. The terrain of the sun-damaged skin is likely to grow more keratoses. Consequently many patients must be treated at regular intervals for this condition.

Another common skin growth that appears on the torso in increasing numbers with aging is the "cherry spot." These pinhead-size clusters of capillaries are benign growths and are generally ignored by both doctor and patient unless unsightly or subject to bleeding. In such cases, they can be removed electrosurgically.

SEBACEOUS CYSTS

A cyst is a saclike structure that is filled with a fluid or semi-solid material. Skin cysts are called *wens* or *sebaceous cysts* or, more properly, *epidermoid cysts*. They are composed of a fibrous wall lined with epithelial cells that produce a cheesy material that forms the contents of the cyst. Wens develop as painless swellings on the back, scalp, or face. When first noted, they may be barely palpable, but they have the potential to gradually enlarge, and occasionally can reach the size of a tennis ball.

Although epidermoid cysts are benign, they not infrequently become infected. Bacteria enter the cyst through a dilated pore that is often visible on the skin surface overlying the cystic

161

swelling. Once inside, the bacteria multiply and the cyst becomes reddened, enlarged, and painful. Badly infected cysts can rupture and discharge pus and the contents of the cyst onto the skin surface. This painful and unpleasant occurrence can sometimes be avoided if the infection is recognized before it progresses to the point where the cyst comes to a head. Early treatment by your dermatologist using warm compresses and an appropriate oral antibiotic, or incision and drainage, can eliminate the infection and return the cyst to its pre-infected appearance.

Treatment One or more episodes of infection are a signal that the cyst should be surgically excised. In fact, it is not a bad idea to have cysts removed before they become infected just to avoid complications later on. The operation consists of opening the skin overlying the cyst, removing the entire sac—preferably in one piece—and closing the incised skin with sutures. Occasionally a cyst will grow back after this procedure if a small remnant of the sac has been left behind.

It should be emphasized that epidermoid cysts are benign growths with little potential to degenerate into skin cancer.

DERMATOFIBROMAS

Often confused with moles, *dermatofibromas* (also called *histiocytomas*) are firm, dark brown nodules that occur most frequently on the lower extremities. In contrast to moles, they grow deeper in the skin and are much firmer since they are composed of fibrous tissue and the cells that make connective tissue. Dermatofibromas may develop after a minor injury such as an insect bite or a hair follicle infection. As such they are more like a localized scar than a tumor. Since they are benign and rarely produce any symptoms, once identified they can be ignored. If they are particularly unsightly or subject to repeated trauma—women often cut them when shaving their legs—they can be surgically excised.

Obviously this discussion of benign skin growths is not all-inclusive. There are dozens more benign growths derived from sweat glands, nerve cells, muscle cells, and all the cells and tissues that make up the skin and the subcutaneous area. But the growths described in this chapter probably constitute 90 percent of the benign growths that are brought to a dermatologist's attention.

13 SKIN PIGMENTATION

Melanocytes are tiny pigment-forming cells that are scattered among the skin cells in the lower epidermis; each is a tiny factory synthesizing a complex dark brown pigment called *melanin*. The melanin is passed on into the epidermal cells that surround each melanocyte. Once "melanized," these epidermal cells remain pigmented throughout their life cycle, and dark melanin granules can be found in all layers of human skin, including the dead surface cells.

In lower animal forms, melanin pigment provides attractive decoration for mating purposes, as well as for camouflage. Certain species of reptiles and amphibians, such as the chameleon and the frog, are capable of changing their color to match their environment in a matter of minutes simply by redistributing the pigment in the skin cells. In human beings its major function is one of protection from the sun. Melanin is uniquely suited to absorb visible and ultraviolet light rays, preventing their penetration into the underlying tissues. As a consequence, heavily pigmented skin is much less likely than pale, nonpigmented skin to suffer from sun damage.

It would be logical to assume that differences of skin color are determined by the number of melanocytes in the skin. The fact is, however, that we all have roughly the same number of pigment-synthesizing cells distributed throughout our skin. Differences in skin color are really determined by the activity of the melanocyte and, more specifically, by the way the melanin is *arranged* inside the epidermal cells after it has been transferred from the melanocyte. In white skin, melanin is aggregated into little packets of granules, while in black skin the pigment is dispersed throughout the cell as single particles. The latter arrangement provides a more light-absorbing surface, and since absorbed light is not reflected back to the viewing eye, the skin appears darker in color.

Although the activity of the melanocyte is determined in part by genetic makeup, there are other factors that can regulate this aspect of cell function. Among the hormonal influences, estrogen, the female hormone, is a stimulant to pigment formation. This pigmenting ability is evident during pregnancy, when there are increased amounts of estrogen in the blood, and a concomitant darkening of the skin around the nipples and an increase in the pigmentation of existing moles.

All forms of radiation are the most important *external* influence on melanocyte activity. Both X ray and heat rays can stimulate pigment formation, but it is ultraviolet and light rays from the sun that provide day-to-day stimulation, resulting in tanning of the skin.

The melanocyte does not always function in a way that is cosmetically pleasing. It can cause conditions of the skin where too much pigment is formed, and others where normal pigment is lacking.

HYPERPIGMENTATION

Any form of inflammation—be it a sunburn, abrasion, or rash—can stimulate the melanocyte to overproduce pigment. When the hyperpigmentation is the result of a prior inflammation, it is reasonable to give it a chance to fade away spontaneously rather than resort to using bleaching creams and lotions.

Melasma

Elevated levels of estrogen hormone in the circulatory system, associated with either pregnancy or the ingestion of an oral contraceptive, can cause an unattractive discoloration on the sun-exposed areas of the face. The term *melasma* has replaced the older term, *chloasma,* and the ugly expression "the mask of pregnancy." Not infrequently, women who are neither pregnant nor on the pill will develop a melasma-like pattern of pigmentation that cannot be explained by a dermatologist or a gynecologist.

Melasma associated with pregnancy often will fade within the year following childbirth. When it occurs with ingestion of an oral contraceptive the prognosis is not quite as good, particularly if the pill is taken for any length of time after the pigmentation becomes apparent. Then excessive sun exposure will darken the already hyperpigmented skin and may lead to a chronic skin condition.

Berloque Dermatitis

Certain perfumes, colognes, after-shave lotions, and other scented cosmetics contain chemicals such as bergamot oil that increase skin sensitivity to sunlight. The perfume or lotion itself will not cause a reaction, but the combination of perfume and sunlight causes a "phototoxic" rash that leaves a striking hyperpigmentation on the skin when it heals. This unusually patterned discoloration appears on the sides of the neck, wrists, and breast cleavage, the usual sites of perfume application. The rash is called *berloque dermatitis,* from the French word meaning "pendant," which aptly describes the droplike shape of the pigmented spots.

There are also a number of plants that can cause similar rashes following prolonged contact with the skin and subsequent exposure to the sun. This condition is called *phytophotodermatitis* and can be caused by lemons, limes, celery, parsnips, and figs, as well as the bergamot (a member of the citrus family) previously mentioned.

Treatment

Once the hyperpigmentation has developed, it is slow to fade and difficult to remove with depigmenting agents. Once again, the most effective treatment is prevention. Since the ingredients of most perfumes and colognes are known only to the manufacturers, it is impossible for you to predict which cosmetics will cause this photosensitization reaction. The solution to the dilemma: "Don't mix sun and scent." Perfume, in various guises, should not be applied if you anticipate a period of sun exposure.

There is an additional reason for you to avoid using scented cosmetics when outdoors in sunny weather: Bees are less likely to be attracted to normal human odor than to perfumes and colognes.

HYPERPIGMENTATION FROM MEDICATION

There are many medications that can alter normal skin color, too. In the past, when syphilis, asthma, anemia, or simply being underweight called for treatment with arsenic, a bronze discoloration of the skin was a sign that large doses of this metal had been consumed. Many years later, patients who had received arsenic as a medication developed multiple skin cancers, another sign of an excessive intake of this metal.

Large doses of silver salts can cause a bluish discoloration of the skin, which is most noticeable in the moons of the nails. Gold salts, still widely used in the treatment of rheumatoid arthritis, can be responsible for excessive amounts of brown pigment around the eyes and on other areas of the skin exposed to light.

During the Second World War, servicemen stationed in the Pacific developed yellow skin because of the regular ingestion of quinacrine and similar drugs that were taken to prevent and treat malaria.

Other medications that cause pigmentation abnormalities include chlorpromazine, a potent tranquilizer; some of the medications used to treat seizure disorders; and a few of the anticancer chemotherapy drugs. But the sum total of these reactions cannot compare with the many pigmentary changes (melasma) experienced by women who take the birth control pill.

Treatment for Hyperpigmentation

As previously noted, the unsightly pigmentation that follows a burn, abrasion, or rash will fade away in a matter of months. In all forms of hyperpigmentation, regardless of the cause, it is usually worthwhile to give nature a chance to repair the damage, especially since the current methods of treatment are not always successful.

People with this problem often turn to over-the-counter medications that are of dubious value and that may sometimes lead to new complications. For example, the cosmetic, nonprescription bleaching creams that are recommended for lightening freckles, melasma, and other forms of excessive pigmentation contain ammoniated mercury, which purportedly blocks the chemical reactions that produce melanin. This sounds fine in theory, but mercury bleaching creams are ineffective, and irritation or allergic reactions can cause you additional distress.

The medical treatment of excessive and undesirable pigmentation is more successful than the cosmetic remedies. The medication most widely prescribed is a chemical called *hydroquinone*. Its discovery was pure chance. Black workers who were handling rubber products containing hydroquinone developed a loss of pigment on their hands and on other areas that were exposed to the chemical. Some time later, the therapeutic application of the chemical that caused this unfortunate reaction was recognized.

Hydroquinone is prescribed as a 1 to 5 percent lotion or salve. Sometimes it is used in combination with retinoic acid to increase penetration into the skin, and a corticosteroid to reduce undesirable irritation. The depigmentation response is erratic at best, and several months of daily application are required in order to determine if it will work at all. Like mercury preparations, hydroquinone can cause irritation or allergic reactions that are severe enough to warrant discontinuation of the treatment, and preparations that are too strong may leave a mottled, unattractive result.

If bleaching fails, then try using a suitable cosmetic that is designed to blend the hyperpigmented area with the surrounding, normally pigmented skin.

TATTOOS

A tattoo is a form of artificial skin pigmentation that is usually acquired by choice. Rarely, an accidental puncture wound will deposit a piece of pencil lead or cinder deep into the skin, creating a limited but permanent tattoo.

The habit and art of tattooing can be traced back to the ancient Egyptians. Mummies have been found with intact skin decorated with tattoos showing animals and religious symbols. Contemporary tattooing is accomplished with an electric needle that deposits colored particles deep in the dermis. The needle passes through the skin with minimal discomfort, depositing, according to preference, black pigment derived from carbon, red pigment in the form of mercury salts, blue pigment from cobalt, or green pigment derived from chrome or iron; when complete, intricate designs, pictures, or words are permanently etched on the skin.

A rare complication from color tattooing can occur if the individual has an allergy to either mercury or chrome. This becomes apparent if the red or green portions of the tattoo become inflamed and swollen. A skin test for the metal will confirm the diagnosis of metal allergy, but treatment is not as simple and may require removal of the tattoo.

Removal of Tattoos

While some tattoos can be removed by surgery, all but the very smallest require a skin graft to close the wound—not a very satisfactory cosmetic solution to the problem. Use of a laser or dermabrasion (see chapter 4) is useful in removing some tattoos, but often the pigment is too deep in the skin to be removed without causing disfiguring scars.

Salabrasion is an interesting and relatively simple technique of tattoo removal, but it is not without its problems. The physician uses a sterile gauze pad dipped into table salt (some prefer the coarse, kosher variety) and vigorously abrades the tattooed area until the skin appears red and glistening, indicating that the epidermis has been removed. The wound is then covered

169

with a dressing that is changed daily. The inflammation produced by the salt and mechanical abrasion dislodges the tattoo
pigment and, over several days, the particles are carried to the
surface and onto the dressings. After the wound heals, the
process can be repeated if necessary. One or more salabrasions
will lighten, if not remove, most tattoos, but like the other methods of tattoo removal, scarring is a potential complication. Of
all the techniques, however, salabrasion is the simplest for altering, if not totally eliminating, large tattoos.

HYPOPIGMENTATION

Burns, abrasions, and rashes that usually heal with an increase
in pigmentation sometimes do just the opposite and turn off
melanocyte function. The end result is pale, depigmented areas
of skin at the site of the inflammation.

In some forms of very mild dermatitis, the signs of irritation
that lead to pigment loss come and go unnoticed, and the problem is not recognized until areas of pale, depigmented skin
appear. This condition is most frequently seen on the face and
upper arms and is referred to as *pityriasis alba*. The unexpected
development of these white spots can be alarming, and suggests
the possibility of a more serious pigmentation disease, *vitiligo*.
Fortunately, normal daily sun exposure (not sunbathing), or
simply the passage of time, will see a restoration of normal
pigmentation to these areas of postinflammatory pigment loss.

Chemically Induced Hypopigmentation

Hydroquinone, a chemical used in rubber products and found
in photographic developer, has caused unexpected depigmentation in some individuals exposed to these products.

Similarly, germicides containing phenol can bleach the skin.
A young man, fastidious in his habits, each day sprayed his
much-used office phone with a phenolic germicide. One day
he noted white spots on his jaw and neck. Fortunately the cause
was identified, and the white areas repigmented spontaneously.

Infections Causing Hypopigmentation

The most common and most innocuous infectious disease that causes pigment loss is *tinea versicolor* (see chapter 9). This superficial fungal infection produces hypopigmented or brown flat spots on the torso and neck. The fungus organism manufactures an acid that interferes with pigment cell function, resulting in diminished pigmentation of the affected areas of skin. If the fungus is eliminated with appropriate treatment, the skin will repigment, although it may take several months to return to normal. In some areas of the world depigmented skin suggests the diagnosis of more serious infections, such as leprosy or yaws.

Albinism

Albinism is fortunately a rare hereditary disease, but it has far-reaching consequences for the individuals afflicted. Albinos are born with a population of melanocytes that is incapable of synthesizing normal quantities of melanin. The signs of this defect are alabaster-white skin, blond to white hair, and an absence of melanin in the normally pigmented portions of the eye. The latter defect is responsible for severe light sensitivity (photophobia) and impaired vision.

Normal amounts of sun exposure can be devastating to albino skin because its major system of sun protection is paralyzed. In primitive societies, where sun exposure was almost unavoidable, death came to middle-aged albinos from skin cancers that were directly related to severe sun-damaged skin cells.

Albinism appears in a milder, more limited form called *piebaldism*. Characteristically, the piebald has a streak of depigmented hair, a white forelock, and scattered patches of white skin. Although piebaldism has cosmetic implications, it is not potentially lethal, as albinism can be.

Vitiligo

While albinos are born with deficient skin pigment, a far more common problem occurs when melanin pigment suddenly dis-

171

appears in childhood or young adulthood, a condition called *vitiligo*. More than one percent of the population will detect white spots on the body during the summertime, when a normal tan makes the vitiliginous areas prominent by contrast. Occasionally, vitiligo will be triggered by a bad sunburn or some other physical stress, but for the most part it appears abruptly and for no apparent reason. The common locations where white spots appear are the back of the hands, the elbows, and the knees, and around the body orifices (mouth, nose, and genitals). Vitiligo may remain limited to a few areas or it may be progressive, with new spots developing and old ones enlarging. Scalp and eyebrow hair can also lose pigment and turn gray, and the body hair that grows out of a vitiliginous patch of skin is almost always white.

The cause of vitiligo is unknown. Although most people with this skin abnormality are in excellent general health, a small number will have an associated systemic illness that is considered to be autoallergic (autoimmune) in origin—that is, their immune system has turned against normal cells in the body. The immune cells, the lymphocytes, attack and destroy tissue in various organs as if these tissues were foreign invaders like bacteria or viruses. Autoallergic diseases are known to affect the thyroid and adrenal glands, the eyes, and even the blood cells. Although it may be guilt by association, the fact that a few people with vitiligo have one of these autoallergic diseases suggests that vitiligo may similarly be the result of the body's immune system gone awry. In this case, the lymphocytes are thought to attack and eventually destroy the melanocytes, thereby eliminating any possibility of pigment formation. Two of the critical questions that remain unanswered by this theory are: What are the factors that incite this peculiar reaction? And why are certain areas of the skin selected for the disease while others go unscathed?

Treatment of Hypopigmentation

Most of the localized pigment loss that follows a rash or injury to your skin will repigment in time if the melanocytes in the area have not been destroyed, as occasionally happens in chemical or thermal burns. In vitiligo, however, spontaneous and complete repigmentation of the white spots is rare.

The chemical psoralen, originally derived from an Egyptian plant, is used by dermatologists in repigmentation therapy. Psoralen sensitizes the skin to ultraviolet light; the combination of this drug and sunlight can stimulate the lethargic melanocyte to manufacture melanin and distribute it to the epidermal cells.

The usual program of treatment requires that you ingest a dose of psoralen medication two hours before ultraviolet light exposure. Since the psoralen increases the skin's reaction to the rays, the initial period of exposure is graded and relatively brief. Subsequent exposures are gradually increased as your tolerance increases.

If the psoralen therapy is successful, new pigment will appear as small spots around hair follicles in the areas of vitiligo. Usually you must undergo months of therapy before there is sufficient repigmentation to be of cosmetic value.

A solution of psoralen can also be applied to the skin to sensitize it to sunlight. This is a less favored method of treatment, since it can cause unpredictable overreaction and severe blistering of the skin. There is also some concern about the long-term consequences of exposure to therapeutic doses of ultraviolet light, particularly the risk of developing skin cancer years later.

The psoralen drugs are available only through prescription, and a program of treatment for vitiligo requires close medical supervision. Many dermatologists are enthusiastic about psoralen therapy, but you should understand that the odds favoring a good cosmetic response are rather poor. Generally, patients with newly acquired vitiligo of less than a year's standing are the ones who will have the best response to treatment. But even a successful psoralen treatment can be followed by relapse and the development of new areas of vitiligo. Psoralen and ultraviolet light are used with a greater degree of success in the treatment of psoriasis (see chapter 3).

As in the treatment of hyperpigmentation, the cosmetic approach would seem to be a reasonable alternative to the use of psoralen. There are several skin dyes, such as the natural juice of black walnuts or the chemical hydroxyacetone, that will satisfactorily mask vitiligo on exposed areas of the body. In severe cases, a skilled cosmetologist can prepare a water-resistant makeup for you that will effectively hide even the most obvious lesions.

14 PEDIATRIC SKIN PROBLEMS

When Mother marches into the doctor's office with Junior in tow, the chances are overwhelming that a skin problem is high on the list of her complaints. It follows that pediatricians who are well versed in their specialty must be knowledgeable in the diagnosis and treatment of skin disorders. Most pediatricians today understand that childhood dermatology requires more than an understanding of adult skin diseases as they might affect younger patients. As in other branches of medicine, the concept that a child is not a miniature adult applies to the skin as well as to the other organs.

Distinctive characteristics of infant skin make it aesthetically pleasing but also susceptible to some unique skin diseases. Some of the anatomical differences are obvious. The skin of a baby is softer, smoother, and virtually hairless as compared to that of an adult. It is dry without being scaly because the immature oil and sweat glands produce little secretion. Newborn infants especially are subject to bodily heat-regulation problems because of their lack of sweat-gland temperature control. As a result, fever not necessarily associated with an illness is not unusual in a newborn during hot weather.

Certain chemical differences in the composition of the small amounts of sweat and oil produced by infantile skin further increase vulnerability to skin infection. And if a baby's skin becomes infected or otherwise inflamed, it tends to respond in

175

a florid manner—with swelling and large blisters—as in the case of impetigo, a streptococcal infection.

INFANTILE ACNE

It is not unusual for newborn babies to have a few whiteheads and pimples on the face. Occasionally this condition can progress to a full-blown case of acne. Fortunately, this is a transient phenomenon, probably related to the effect of the maternal hormones that are transmitted from mother to infant during pregnancy.

Infantile acne may be upsetting to the parents, but the blemishes don't bother the baby at all. No treatment is necessary since the outbreak is temporary. Above all, it should be understood that infantile acne is *not* a harbinger of acne or other skin problems in adult life.

Small yellow or white pimples on the eyelids, forehead, and cheeks of the baby are an equally common infantile blemish. These lesions, called *milia,* are the result of the blockage of an oil gland duct close to the surface of the skin. Like the acne lesions, milia disappear without any treatment.

HEAT RASH

Infants and young children are singularly susceptible to the blockage of the ducts that transport fluid from the sweat glands to the surface of the skin. The appearance of the resulting heat rash, or *miliaria,* depends on the level at which the sweat ducts become occluded. Obstruction close to the skin surface creates many tiny superficial blisters. The appearance of hundreds of these glistening vesicles suggests the descriptive name, *miliaria crystallina.* This mildest form of heat rash requires no treatment since the blisters spontaneously break and peel off, reopening the blocked sweat ducts.

When blockage occurs deeper in the duct, there is a combination of blisters and small red bumps associated with a distinctive itching and stinging sensation. This form of heat rash is appropriately called "prickly heat," and can occur in both children and adults.

Heat rashes of all types occur in a hot, humid environment. They are common in the summertime but may pass unrecognized at other times of the year. For example, infants who are dressed in multiple layers of clothing may fall victim to a winter form of heat rash.

Treatment

The key to the treatment of all forms of miliaria is establishing a cool, low-humidity environment. Air-conditioning is helpful, if available. An attempt should be made to keep the infant's skin dry with cornstarch, baby powder, or a cooling lotion made up of equal amounts of witch hazel and rubbing alcohol. Avoid the use of thick creams or lotions that merely increase the blockage of the sweat ducts and add to the problem.

DIAPER RASH

Diaper rash is undoubtedly the most common and vexing skin problem of infancy. Almost every baby will have some signs of irritation in the diaper area at one time or another, but the severity may vary from a faint redness that disappears without special care or medication, to a blistering or pustular rash that defies all forms of treatment. Parents are justifiably vexed when they learn that the medical profession is unable to agree on the specific cause of simple diaper rash. The theories that have been proposed are as varied as the pet treatments of pediatricians and dermatologists who deal with the problem daily.

There is general agreement that the most important causal factor is the warm, moist environment characteristic of the diaper region. This humid environment leads to a persistent irritation called *intertrigo*, which occurs when skin surfaces oppose each other and aeration and evaporation are inhibited. In ad-

177

dition to intertrigo, the presence of bacteria, fungus, ammonia, soap, detergents, as well as other skin diseases such as seborrheic or contact dermatitis, play a variable role in the origin of diaper rash.

Many pediatricians believe that ammonia is the crux of the diaper rash problem. It is well known that skin bacteria living in the diaper region can manufacture ammonia from the urea present in the urine. Proponents of the ammonia theory believe that neutralizing this chemical with an acid, or killing the bacteria that produce this chemical, will prevent diaper rash. To this end, some doctors prescribe a medication to acidify the urine while others recommend that the diapers be washed in vinegar or commercial rinses that inhibit bacterial growth. Physicians who disagree with this approach point to the fact that the ammonia concentration that is found in the diapers is not strong enough to irritate normal skin. Furthermore, a strong ammonia odor and a high concentration of ammonia in diapers are found in many infants who never experience significant diaper dermatitis.

Infections by bacteria and by the fungus *Candida albicans* can complicate diaper rash. The diaper area provides an ideal environment for these organisms to multiply and infect the skin. Treatment with an antibiotic or antifungal ointment prescribed by a physician will occasionally clear the diaper rash completely.

Treatment

The fact that there are so many different treatments of diaper dermatitis confirms the obvious: There is no panacea for this common disease. The general measures that are recommended by most doctors are at least as important as the medication selected to be applied to the inflamed skin. These therapeutic maneuvers include the elimination of plastic pants, the avoidance of soap, a switch to cloth diapers and away from disposable diapers (some babies are allergic to the plastic lining, and the plastic can enhance the humidity in which bacteria thrive), a change in diaper detergent or rinse, and exposing the skin to encourage aeration and drying. In severe cases of diaper rash, simply eliminate the diaper altogether until the rash clears up.

This method may be messy, but it often works when other treatments fail.

When it comes to selecting a topical medication, a heavy, protective ointment is fine for mild diaper rash, but it may aggravate the condition if a bacterial or fungal infection is present. Nystatin, miconazole, and amphotericin B and other antifungal agents are prescribed for fungal infection, and bacitracin, neomycin, and triple antibiotic ointments are recommended for a bacterial infection.

The persistent use of corticosteroid ointments or creams to reduce redness and the other signs of irritation is rarely necessary and can have an adverse effect on the thin and vulnerable skin of the diaper area.

SEBORRHEIC DERMATITIS OF INFANCY

"Cradle cap," the familiar yellowish, scaling rash on baby's scalp, is the mildest and most common form of infantile seborrheic dermatitis. In the more severe cases, the rash spreads to the face, the torso, and the diaper area. Unlike infants with allergic eczema who scratch and tear at their itchy skin, babies with seborrheic dermatitis appear unaffected by the rash.

Both the adult and infant forms of seborrheic dermatitis remain on the list of diseases of unknown cause, although there may be a genetic predisposition to the condition. In contrast to the chronic and recurring adult form, infantile seborrheic dermatitis invariably disappears around the time of the child's first birthday.

Treatment

Given the limited duration of the problem, treatment should be restrained since medications are not curative and time is the ultimate healer. You can treat cradle cap with an overnight application of baby oil, or with a mild ointment containing a small amount of salicyclic acid, which will soften the adhering scales. A morning shampoo with ordinary baby shampoo or one of the mild commercial dandruff shampoos will help to remove the scales. Body lesions will improve with the use of ointments containing sulfur (not sulfa). The use of topical steroids on children's skin is not recommended. Corticosteroids should be used only if necessary, and with great caution, because of the risk of thinning of the skin as well as of systemic side effects.

IMPETIGO

Infants and young children are susceptible to most of the same infectious diseases as adults, and often to a greater degree. In addition to the anatomical features that make babies' skin especially vulnerable to infection, the immature immune system affords reduced protection against many infectious germs.

Impetigo is a superficial bacterial skin infection. Newborns are very susceptible to a severe form of this disease caused by staphylococcus bacteria. The infected skin becomes covered with yellowish blisters that break and peel off, leaving moist, reddened areas denuded of epidermis. The blistering form of impetigo is extremely contagious, and if proper precautions are not followed, the infection is easily transmitted from baby to baby in the hospital nursery, or from baby to mother or to other family members at home. Most hospital nurseries follow rigid antiseptic procedures to prevent impetigo and other infections; masks and gowns are the rule, and personnel or visitors with any form of infection are forbidden entry. If a baby develops any signs of this or any other contagious disease, he or she is quickly isolated from the other infants.

Impetigo in older children and adults is less dramatic. The infection starts when the streptococcus bacteria, with or without their traveling companions the staphylococci, enter through a small opening in the skin surface. Although the impetigo sore may form on what appears to be healthy skin, it more often occurs as a complication of minor cuts, insect bites, squeezed pimples, or fever blisters. These slowly healing sores are frequently ignored or incorrectly treated for days before the correct medical diagnosis is made. It is often the appearance of new blisters with yellowish scabs on other parts of the body that points to the infectious nature of the skin rash.

Acute glomerulonephritis, a disease of the kidneys, is a rare but serious complication of streptococcal impetigo. Certain strains of the streptococcus bacteria stimulate the immune system to form antibodies that inflame the kidneys. The first signs of nephritis—swelling of the face and legs (edema) and blood in the urine—do not appear until several weeks after the skin infection has healed. It remains questionable whether early treatment of the impetigo will prevent nephritis from occurring in children who are susceptible to this disease.

Treatment

To some extent, the therapy for impetigo depends upon its severity. The traditional treatment of one or two small areas of infection has been to bathe the infected skin with soap and water to soften and remove the crust, and to apply an antibiotic ointment containing bacitracin, erythromycin, or some other antibiotic that is active against streptococcal bacteria. Studies of treated and untreated impetigo suggest that locally applied antibiotics do not necessarily speed up the rate of healing. There is no question, however, that antibiotics administered orally or by injection will cure impetigo rapidly and completely. In recent years, the trend has been to treat this infection with a systemic antibiotic in all but the very mildest cases.

BIRTHMARKS

There are discolorations and marks on a newborn's skin that are the result of a rough passage through the birth canal. These are "birthmarks" in the true sense of the word. Invariably, these transient bumps and bruises disappear during the first few weeks of life. More permanent birthmarks are alterations of skin pigmentation or blood vessel growths that are actually developmental abnormalities and are unrelated to events that occur at the time of birth.

Mongolian Spot

The *Mongolian spot* is the most common pigmentary change in black and oriental babies and is not uncommon in white infants. Mongolian spots are flat, blue marks that are found on the middle of the lower back or on the buttocks. These discolorations have absolutely no health significance and usually fade away in early childhood.

Epidermal Nevi

Pigmented growths (*nevi*) that are persistent may be of greater concern. They are derived from two different sources. The cells of the epidermis can form birthmarks that first appear as flat, brown streaks or lines. As the baby matures, these epidermal moles become more obvious as the spots and lines become elevated and acquire a rough and irregular surface.

These kinds of pigmented epidermal birthmarks have no tendency to change into malignant growths, and they deserve attention only if they are unsightly, or if their location on the body causes physical discomfort. It is a judgment call on the part of the physician and parents whether or not to remove the birthmark early in the life of the child, or to wait until the child is old enough to participate in the decision-making process and to cooperate at the time of surgical removal. Some physicians feel that the younger the child, the smaller the incision and the smaller the resulting scar. Each decision to operate must be judged on a case-by-case basis.

Congenital Moles

Pigmented birthmarks derived from melanocytes, the pigment-forming cells, can be present at birth. These *congenital* moles (nevi) are believed to have a greater potential to undergo malignant change into melanoma than are the acquired nevi, the flat, brown-to-black moles that first begin to appear in early childhood (see chapter 12).

Hemangiomas

Birthmarks that are composed of blood vessels are called *hemangiomas*. The mildest ones appear as faint areas of redness on the eyelids and on the back of the neck at the time of birth. These so-called salmon patches usually fade away before the first birthday. The more persistent, flat type of hemangioma, called the *nevus flammeus* or port-wine stain, is dark red, at times almost black in color and usually appears on one side of the face.

Methods of treatment of this form of hemangioma are not particularly satisfactory. Small port-wine hemangiomas can be removed surgically, but this is not a practical approach for the large hemangiomas that cover the side of the face or most of a limb. In recent years the laser has been used successfully to treat some of these lesions.

In contrast to the flat, port-wine hemangioma, the strawberry mark, or *capillary hemangioma,* is an elevated, soft, red growth of capillaries that is present at birth or appears on the skin during the early months of life. This form of blood-vessel growth enlarges rapidly during the first few years of life but then shrinks in size, in most instances disappearing with little residual scarring. Although it may take years for capillary hemangiomas to clear up, by age seven more than 75 percent of these birthmarks will have disappeared without any treatment.

Treatment

Physicians who are familiar with the spontaneous resolution of most hemangiomas usually recommend watchful waiting for most birthmarks rather than undertaking a form of treatment that may cause more scarring than does the natural, self-healing process. In rare instances where the hemangioma interferes with eating or breathing—a situation that occurs when large, expanding growths exist around the nose and mouth—treatment is necessary and cannot be withheld. If surgical removal is not practical, there are other modes of treatment, such as laser surgery, radiation, freezing, or the administration of corticosteroid drugs. But all forms of treatment for this problem

183

carry some degree of risk, including the formation of disfiguring scars from freezing or laser surgery, side effects from corticosteroids, or the long-term damage to the skin from radiation.

It is worth repeating that treatment can and should be withheld in most cases.

RASHES AND FEVERS

The sudden appearance of a rash and a high fever in a child can be an alarming and puzzling problem to parents and physicians alike. Even with sophisticated laboratory tests, the pediatrician or family doctor may not be able to diagnose the illness immediately. Today it has become increasingly difficult to sort out all of the infectious diseases that cause a fever and a rash. And, while modern techniques of studying viruses and other infectious organisms have expanded medical knowledge, in a sense a number of "new" diseases have been exposed.

Since the list of febrile rashes is already long and continuously growing, the illnesses considered in this section include some of the traditional rashes of childhood, several of the viral diseases that are distinctive and relatively easy to identify, and a few diseases the causes of which remain unknown.

Measles

Widespread immunization with vaccine over the past few decades has all but eliminated the once-common virus infection of measles (*rubeola*). From time to time, a new case will turn up among youngsters and adults who somehow failed to receive their immunization. The measles rash is preceded by a high fever and the three Cs familiar to all medical students—a cough, a cold, and conjunctivitis (inflammation of the eyes). Red spots with a white center on the cheeks inside of the mouth (Koplik spots) are another early sign of measles that precedes the body rash.

After several days of the coldlike illness, a red, papular rash appears behind the ears and spreads down the neck to the trunk and finally to the extremities. The rash takes three to four days to evolve and, after another week, the spots turn brown and scaly and peeling occurs. Since there is no antiviral agent active against the measles virus, treatment is limited to rest, acetaminophen for the fever (aspirin is not recommended for children because of the danger of Reye's syndrome), dark glasses for eye discomfort, and cough medicine if necessary.

German Measles

Although *rubella,* or German measles, is a mild illness in children and adults, it does have serious implications if acquired by a woman during the early weeks of pregnancy. The rubella virus can infect the developing fetus and cause stillbirth or serious congenital abnormalities. An effective vaccine is now available, and these complications can be avoided if a woman is immunized early in her life, years before childbearing age.

German measles develop after a two- to three-week incubation period. A low-grade fever and mild symptoms of a cold precede the pink, papular rash that appears on the face and spreads to the entire body within a twenty-four-hour period. Often large, tender lymph glands can be palpated on the back of the neck before the rash apears. Rubella lasts only two to three days and confers permanent immunity against further infections with the virus.

Chicken Pox

Chicken pox, or *varicella,* is composed of small blisters arising on reddened skin—the rash has been described quite poetically as appearing like "dew drops on a rose petal." Most of the blemishes appear on the torso, with a few blisters appearing on the extremities, face, scalp, and inside of the mouth. Outbreaks of new lesions occur for three to four days, and it takes close to three weeks for complete healing. Chicken pox can cause permanent scars particularly if the healing crusts are removed prematurely, or if a bacterial infection develops in the pox blisters.

185

Since chicken pox can be a more serious illness for older children and adults, and is sometimes accompanied by a high fever and pneumonia, most physicians believe it is just as well to "get over" chicken pox in early childhood. There is no vaccine that will prevent chicken pox, and no special antiviral treatment once infection occurs. Individuals whose immune response to the virus has been paralyzed by disease or by immunosuppressive drugs have been treated with the antiviral agent acyclovir, in an attempt to prevent the most severe complications of chicken pox infection.

The same virus that causes chicken pox is responsible for herpes zoster (shingles), a painful, blistering rash that follows the path of a spinal nerve root (see chapter 9).

Scarlet Fever

Some strains of streptococcus bacteria secrete a chemical that causes the rash of scarlet fever. The illness starts with headache, fever, and a very sore throat. After a few days, a red flush appears on the neck and chest, and a fine pebbly rash spreads from the face to the rest of the body. Since the rash of scarlet fever can be easily confused with some of the viral diseases, check for red streaks in the folds of the elbows and knees, pallor around the mouth and the tip of the nose, and a swollen and red "strawberry" tongue—all findings that are a tip-off to the correct diagnosis.

Treatment Scarlet fever is a bacterial rather than a viral infection and responds to treatment with antibiotics. The streptococcus bacterium is particularly sensitive to penicillin. In the case of an allergic reaction (hives, rash) to that antibiotic, erythromycin or one of the other antibiotics that act against streptococci can be substituted by your doctor.

Roseola Infantum

A high fever (102 to 106 degrees) lasting up to five days precedes the rash of roseola. During the febrile phase of the illness parents and physician are likely to worry about all sorts of serious diseases that might be responsible for the fever. All parties concerned are greatly relieved when the fever falls abruptly and a measles-like rash appears on the body and, to a lesser extent, on the arms and legs. The rash of roseola subsides within a day or two without any treatment.

Hand, Foot, and Mouth Disease

A summer illness that affects only human beings, hand, foot, and mouth disease is caused by several strains of the Coxsackie virus, a virus originally isolated in the town of Coxsackie, New York. In addition to hand, foot, and mouth disease, the Coxsackie group of viruses are the cause of a number of other acute illnesses, several of which are associated with skin rashes.

You can recognize hand, foot, and mouth disease by the presence of scattered, painful blisters on the hands, feet, inside of the mouth, and occasionally elsewhere on the body. A sore throat and low-grade fever can accompany the blisters, which heal without treatment within a few days. Hand, foot, and mouth disease is usually a mild illness, but it can be puzzling to parents and doctors not familiar with its unusual manifestations.

Fifth Disease

Fifth disease, or *erythema infectiosum*, is another viral illness that challenges diagnostic skill more than it impairs health. The first sign of this disease is a facial flush that creates a "slapped cheek" appearance. Although the facial redness fades after a few days, a new rash appears on the arms and legs. The second rash is composed of bright red spots that overlap to form a lacy network. This reticulated pattern tends to fade and reappear for many days before it finally disappears.

The rash of fifth disease occurs in children and young adults. At times it is so mild that it passes entirely unnoticed and is diagnosed only retrospectively.

Infectious Mononucleosis

"Mono," as it is familiarly called by young people, can produce a collection of diverse symptoms including fatigue, headache, sore throat, fever, swollen glands, painful joints, and inflammation of the liver. In mono, rashes occur infrequently and they are usually short-lived; they take the appearance of a mild case of German measles or hives. One-third of mono sufferers will have blood spots inside the mouth on the palate that can be a clue to the diagnosis of this viral illness.

Pityriasis Rosea

It is questionable whether *pityriasis rosea* should be included in a discussion of common rashes and fevers. Pityriasis rosea is not a febrile illness, nor has any infectious cause been determined. On the other hand, cases appear to be clustered and possibly seasonal, and to many physicians the pattern of the rash suggests a viral illness.

Pityriasis rosea occurs in adults as well as children and the rash has the same characteristic features. A solitary, round, red, scaly spot, often mistaken for ringworm, is the first sign of the impending eruption. After several days, sometimes weeks, this "herald patch" is followed by a mildly itchy outbreak of many similar but smaller spots on the torso and the upper portions of the arms and legs. On the back, the rash follows the oblique lines of the normal skin folds, producing a linear arrangement of spots that has been likened to the boughs of a Christmas tree. New spots continue to appear for two to three weeks, and an additional two to three weeks elapse before the skin becomes clear.

Pityriasis rosea causes no symptoms other than mild itching. Treatment consists of a doctor's explanation of the disease and a bland anti-itch cream or lotion. It was originally thought that one attack conveyed immunity, but it has become increasingly apparent that some individuals can suffer two or more episodes of this common but poorly understood rash.

Kawasaki Disease

Originally seen in Japan, *Kawasaki disease* has now spread around the globe. Also called the *mucocutaneous lymph node syndrome,* the illness starts with fever and swollen lymph glands in the neck. Subsequently, the eyes become reddened and a rash appears on the body. The rash is variable in its appearance and tends to change from day to day. More distinctive signs include bright, red, tender swelling of the palms and soles, reddening and splitting of the lips, and a swollen, red "strawberry" tongue. The more serious internal manifestations of this disease are not consistent but include meningitis, inflammation of the liver and gallbladder, and heart problems.

Treatment The cause of Kawasaki disease has yet to be identified; hence there is no specific treatment available. Aspirin is recommended to prevent some of the complications associated with heart inflammation.

15 THE PSYCHE AND THE SKIN

From the physician's (and patient's) point of view, the emotions can often serve as a convenient explanation for the origin of otherwise inexplicable skin ailments. Unfortunately, there are still many diseases, in all branches of medicine, that fit into the "cause unknown" category.

There are other reasons for linking the emotions and the skin. Unlike the liver and the kidneys, the skin is only too visible. Since contemporary society places a high value on physical appearance, many anxious people tend to connect their emotional state with their minor skin problems. In general, however, there is no substantive evidence to support this conclusion.

Of course, it is undeniable that a few skin conditions are genuinely influenced by nervous tension or emotional distress. The skin has an abundant supply of blood vessels and sweat glands that are controlled by the autonomic nervous system— that part of the nervous system that is directly affected by our emotions. Since blood vessels and, to a lesser extent, sweat glands, play an important role in many skin diseases, it is not surprising that stress can at times trigger or worsen an existing skin condition.

In this chapter we will explore some skin disorders that are directly influenced by the emotions, as well as a few others in which the emotions are the chief causal factor.

ACNE ROSACEA

As the name would imply, *acne rosacea* is a red-colored rash. It appears gradually on the cross-shaped "flush" area of the face—the cheeks, nose, midforehead, and chin—an area distinctive for its many small blood vessels that are sensitive to stimulation and dilatation from foods, drugs, and temperature changes as well as the emotions. Individuals who develop acne rosacea appear to have a supersensitive group of blood vessels that dilate more readily than normal and fail to completely return to their normal constricted state after the flush-provoking stimulus has been removed.

After years of this exaggerated blood-vessel behavior, a persistent flush and tiny veins appear on the skin surface. Finally, in many patients with this disorder, acne-like blemishes erupt on the red skin.

Acne rosacea is clearly not a psychosomatic disease; rather, it is an unexplained disorder of the blood vessels that happen to be extremely sensitive to emotional stimulation. Most patients with acne rosacea are aware that an upsetting situation will further brighten their already red face, and they will do their utmost to avoid this form of provocation. In general, tranquilizers are not very effective in treating rosacea unless there happens to be an independent problem of chronic anxiety, and even then the rash is not very responsive to this form of treatment.

Diet has been a traditional form of therapy for acne rosacea, and logically so. Since heat dilates the blood vessels, very hot foods such as steaming cups of coffee, tea, or soup, or very spicy foods are taboo. Alcohol is another potent vasodilator that should be consumed in limited quantities. The concept that alcohol is the cause of rosacea and of the swollen, red nose that may accompany this ailment, is a false one. At worst, heavy alcohol consumption is an aggravating factor, but many teetotalers suffer from acne rosacea and the red-nose syndrome.

In addition to diet and a look at the psyche, there are only a few medications that can favorably influence the course of this disease. The redness of the skin can be temporarily blanched with corticosteroid creams, but these are not recommended since overuse may actually encourage some of the permanent skin changes of acne rosacea. The acne-like eruptions can be treated with many of the same medications that are used to treat regular acne. The tetracycline antibiotics are particularly effective in eliminating the unsightly pustules and red pimples that often appear suddenly and unexpectedly in this disease. The recent development of a new external medication called *metronidazole gel* is a promising advancement in the treatment of acne rosacea.

Dilated veins on the face can also be eliminated, with good cosmetic results, through a process called *electrodesiccation*. This type of electrosurgery delivers a weak electric current into the blood vessel, damaging its inner wall and shutting it down.

There are other skin diseases in which sensitive or abnormal blood vessels may become subject to emotional influences. Several of these, including urticaria (hives), psoriasis, eczema, and seborrheic dermatitis, are discussed in other chapters.

EXCESSIVE SWEATING

The sweat glands are a temperature-regulating system that permits the dissipation of body heat that we build up through vigorous physical activity or exposure to a hot environment. In addition to heat, the thinking part of the brain can also activate the sweat glands.

Excessive sweating, called *hyperhidrosis,* can be both an embarrassing and incapacitating problem. Moist, dripping palms can be as much of a handicap to a salesman as cystic acne is to an actor or a model. Constant, heavy sweating in the axillary (armpit) area is also an embarrassing and uncomfortable disability that can also damage underclothes and outer garments.

Why do some people perspire to this unpleasant extent? Are they all high-strung, nervous individuals? Not necessarily. There are tense individuals who sweat excessively, but many of the most severe "oversweaters" are not hyperemotional. In fact, when they do appear nervous, it is often a circular response to their concern about excessive perspiration rather than vice versa.

All of this suggests that the defect is not in the mind, but somewhere in the nervous system's sweat-gland control mechanism. Minimal heat or emotional stimulation turns on the sweat glands full throttle. The nerves may be overstimulating the glands, or the glands may be responding to the stimulation in an excessive and uncontrolled manner. The problem can be compared to a broken-down thermostat. The setting is normal or low but the furnace continues to fire away.

Treatment

Most people who suffer from hyperhidrosis need medical help, not psychotherapy. Tranquilizers that tone down the nerve impulses to the sweat glands are not very effective in diminishing emotional sweating, and they have the disadvantage of toning down other nervous-system functions as well. A salesman with wet hands doesn't want to feel lethargic or depressed as well.

Other drugs that can block the nervous stimulation of the sweat glands have even more unpleasant side effects at the high dosages required to reduce oversweating. Most heavy perspirers are not keen about trading off this problem for dizziness, a dry mouth, or a difficulty in urination.

The most satisfactory therapy for hyperhidrosis has been achieved through the prescription and use of super-strong antiperspirants, such as 20 percent aluminum chloride in a pure alcohol solution. This chemical can be applied to the underarm area, palms, or soles of the feet overnight and covered with a plastic wrap dressing. Two or three nights of treatment will markedly diminish the sweating, but irritation of the skin may occasionally complicate the results of the treatment. If the medication can be tolerated, further application once or twice a week may maintain sweating at acceptable levels.

At times, excessive sweating of the palms and feet is associated with a blistering rash in these areas. This condition is called *dyshidrosis*, which means "difficult or abnormal sweating." A theory that has not been confirmed by scientific studies is that the tiny, very itchy blisters that develop deep in the palms and feet are the result of a blockage of the sweat gland ducts. True or not, most patients with dyshidrosis seem to feel that the worst blistering occurs at times of emotional crisis, and so dyshidrosis has been considered by some to be on the fringe of psychosomatic ailments.

As in simple oversweating, the blistering rash of dyshidrosis does not respond to treatment with tranquilizers or other techniques for "cooling off." Most dermatologists will treat this problem with the general methods used to treat all forms of dermatitis.

ITCHING

Unexplained itching, *pruritus,* is one of the most common symptoms attributed to psychological factors. But itching over the entire body without signs of a rash can be caused by many illnesses that should be considered and investigated before accepting a simple diagnosis of "nervous itch."

Elderly people, for instance, experience widespread itching in the wintertime because their skin becomes dry. There may be no evidence of a rash, but the severe itching will abate with lubrication, a reduction in bathing, and an increase in environmental humidity.

There are also a number of systemic illnesses that cause widespread itching. Itching without a rash is a clue to a disease that may not have been previously recognized. Diabetes and various diseases that affect the liver can be heralded by unexplained itching. The itch list also includes kidney ailments, internal cancer, and thyroid disease. Some medications can initiate itching, though most reactions to medications do cause rash along with the itch.

A number of patients suffer from persistent itching although they do not have any detectable illness that might explain away the problem. Not all of these individuals should be considered to have a nervous disorder; however, it is equally important not to deny the fact that extreme itching can be an emotional symptom, indicating depression or a similar mental condition.

Other, more localized forms of itching may be influenced by the mind. Persistent itching of the genital skin or the skin around the anus is an annoying symptom that can interfere with sleep as well as normal social activities. The emotional distress produced by the itch tends to obscure the fact that psychosexual factors may be exacerbating the problem. The paroxysmal bouts of itching followed by scratching in these erogenous areas produces a pattern of sensation that has been compared to orgasm.

But it is also important not to overlook other possible causes of itching in the anal and genital areas, including such problems as fungal infection, pinworm infestations, allergic reactions, psoriasis, and poor hygiene. These possibilities should be considered *before* turning to the psyche, which offers a not easily validated explanation for these symptoms.

Another form of localized itching can lead to a thickened, red, scaly patch of irritated skin at the site of persistent scratching. This condition is called *neurodermatitis* and it can be best explained by what has been called the "itch-scratch cycle." A localized skin irritation may initiate the itching. The reflex scratching magnifies the irritation and stimulates the sensitive nerve endings, which send out more messages of itch. The cycle of scratching producing more itching continues long after the cause of the original irritation has disappeared. Eventually, the affected skin becomes an island of dermatitis that is continuously sending out scratch-provoking signals that perpetuate the problem. Some people use scratching as a tension-release mechanism, so although they are willing to face up to the fact that the skin problem is self-induced, they are incapable of resisting the impulse to scratch. This is particularly true at night, when they are in a state of half-sleep and not in complete control of their actions.

Treatment

Treatment of neurodermatitis is usually successful if you understand the itch-scratch cycle and accept responsibility for the origin and the persistence of the dermatitis. A corticosteroid cream applied to the irritated skin and covered with a bandage relieves the itching and protects the area from further scratch damage. You can supplement this external treatment with an oral antihistamine or anti-itch tranquilizer at bedtime. These medications will help you get through the night without further intolerable itching.

HAIR PULLING

Pulling out your hair on a chronic basis is another psychocutaneous symptom that may indicate emotional disturbances of greater or lesser severity. Some severely disturbed patients in psychiatric hospitals may pull out their body and scalp hair as a symptom of their mental disease, but hair pulling in most cases is a less serious tension-release phenomenon.

Children, more than adults, will pull or twist their scalp hair, or pull on eyelashes or eyebrows while they are reading or concentrating on other things. Once the child and parent become aware of this habit, the problem can usually be solved. In other youngsters, the compulsive hair-pulling habit indicates an emotional disturbance that may be temporary and is often related to specific events in their lives.

SKIN INFESTATION PHOBIAS AND DELUSIONS

A sensation of being infested with crawling things (*formication*) is not uncommon. Many perfectly normal people will start to itch, or experience creeping sensations, at the very mention of insects or lice. This distress, however, is carried to the extreme by some emotionally disturbed individuals who have actual delusions that they are infested with bugs. These people often tell bizarre tales about tiny creatures that crawl under their skin and infest their furniture and bedclothes. Sometimes, the crawling things are "too small to be visible." But other victims of this delusion often present to the physician an envelope or carefully wrapped tissue that contains the "dead insects" that have been picked off their skin. On close scrutiny, this evidence of the infestation proves to be pieces of dried skin and other debris.

It is virtually impossible for the dermatologist to convince these patients that they are not infested, and "treating" the mythical infestation is never successful. Invariably these distraught people have already visited several physicians who have tried the same approach. Psychiatric help is the obvious answer, if the physician can convince the patient or the family to seek such help.

16 DERMATOLOGICAL COSMETIC PROCEDURES

In the past decade, dermatologists have expanded their interest and expertise in the area of cosmetic surgery. Some of the techniques to be described here may overlap into the field of plastic surgery. Others remain largely in the province of the dermatologist. Most of the procedures are *minor* in the sense that they can be performed in the doctor's office under local anesthesia. Several of the procedures are *major* because of their cosmetic consequences. It is important for the patient to be aware of the risks and complications of cosmetic surgery as well as its potential benefits.

LASERS

Lasers are instruments that produce high-energy light of a very specific wavelength. Laser beams will pass through some tissues of the body and be absorbed by others. When the light energy is absorbed, it turns into heat. In treating certain eye diseases, for instance, a laser beam can be selected that passes through the lens and cornea to reach the pigmented layer of the retina in the back of the eye, where the heat energy of the laser beam will repair tears and other retinal problems.

In the field of dermatology the laser is being used to treat an increasing number of skin disorders that have previously gone untreated or have been treated by other means. The argon laser produces a blue-green ray that is absorbed by melanin pigment and the hemoglobin in red blood cells. Thus it is useful in lightening or eliminating blood vessel growths, such as the birthmarks called port-wine stains. Similarly, pigmented growths such as moles, brown spots, and some tattoos can also be removed with little damage to the surrounding skin.

The carbon dioxide laser is a more versatile instrument because it produces a beam that is absorbed by water. Since the skin is largely made up of water, the energy is absorbed by the superficial layers of the skin. This laser beam can be used in several ways. It can be focused onto a small area and its energy used to cut tissue like a scalpel—the heat of the beam sealing off the blood vessels, resulting in relatively bloodless surgery. The beam can also be used to vaporize tissue, a technique often used to destroy warts and other skin growths.

The cost and maintenance of a laser ranges from $25,000 up to $100,000. Since this is a major investment, some physicians feel obliged to use it to treat conditions that might very well be treated with some other, less expensive surgical modality. This is not to deny that the laser has a unique advantage in treating lesions that are inaccessible to other surgical methods, or where very precise, localized destruction or cutting is desired. Complications from laser surgery are on a par with complications from other surgical techniques.

ELECTROSURGERY

The electrosurgical unit is a standard piece of equipment in almost all dermatologists' offices. The laser may very well be the instrument of the future, but for the present electrosurgery is a more versatile and much less expensive technique. Like the laser the electrosurgical unit can be used to cut, to destroy tissue, and to seal severed blood vessels to control bleeding.

Among the more delicate operations frequently performed with electrosurgery, dilated veins on the face (due to chronic sun damage or a disease called *acne rosacea*, see page 191) can be eliminated with good cosmetic results through a process called *electrodesiccation*. A fine needle is used to deliver a weak electric current into the blood vessel, damaging its inner wall and shutting it down. Similarly, spider angiomas, which are dilated blood vessels with spider leg–like appendages, can be destroyed electrosurgically without significant scarring. Other lesions that lend themselves to treatment with electrosurgery include liver spots, small cysts, keratoses, warts, and some forms of skin cancer.

SCLEROTHERAPY

This injection technique is designed to treat small varicosities, sometimes called "sunburst veins," that commonly occur on the legs. These dilated veins are larger in caliber than the fine veins that occur on the face and that are amenable to electrosurgical destruction.

Sclerotherapy involves inserting a very fine needle into the major vein of a sunburst plexus and injecting a concentrated salt solution, or some other chemical that causes irritation of the lining of the major vein and veins that branch off of it. Subsequently, through the formation of either a clot or a scar, the small veins shrink down and fade away.

The results, however, cannot be guaranteed. Sometimes several injection sessions are required to eliminate an area of interconnecting veins. The most common side effect of sclerotherapy is the appearance of pigmented spots in the skin thought to be due to the leakage of blood at the injection sites. These are usually temporary and fade after several months. Occasionally permanent depressed scars develop if the sclerosing solution leaks out of the vein into the surrounding tissues. But, by and large, this is a safe procedure with no serious side effects.

LIPOSUCTION

Remodeling the body's contours by removing fat deposits has become the number-one cosmetic surgical procedure in the

United States, surpassing the face-lift in popularity. The procedure can be done because fat cells do not regenerate after destruction or removal, as evidenced by the fact that individuals who gain weight after liposuction do not regain significant amounts of weight in areas of previous fat removal.

Liposuction is accomplished by inserting a tube called a *canula* through a small incision in the skin. The tube, attached to a suction pump, is forcibly moved through the fat, disrupting and removing the fat cells. The vigorous movement of the canula produces tunnels in the fat that scar down, resulting in a permanent flattening of the area treated. Ultimate improvement does not occur until the scarring process is complete. After surgery the patient may experience soreness and notice black-and-blue discolorations due to bleeding under the skin. Occasionally, bleeding during liposuction can be excessive and it becomes necessary to interrupt or discontinue the procedure.

The localized fat deposits that are the favorite targets of the liposuctionist are the fat deposits on the flanks, the buttocks, the abdomen, and fatty areas around the knees and ankles, and under the chin. Many of these liposuction operations are performed under local anesthesia in the doctor's office. Complications include excessive bleeding and shock reactions. Also, unless scrupulously sterile techniques are used, infection may occur. Radical fat removal is radical surgery, and requires hospitalization and general anesthesia, with all its attendant risks.

The most frequent cosmetic side effect of liposuction is a ridging of the skin surface—an external reflection of the tunnels created in the fat deposit by the surgical procedure. Although ridging may be unsightly when the patient is nude or in a bathing suit, it is not apparent when he or she is fully dressed.

SKIN PEELS

Skin peels are most effective when used to modify the superficial lines, furrows, and discolorations associated with chronic sun damage. The peeling agent, usually phenol or trichloroacetic acid, is applied to the skin with cotton-tipped applicator sticks.

The concentration of these caustic agents will determine the depth of the peel. Taping of the skin after the chemical has been applied increases penetration and thus the depth of the peel.

After the peeling agent has been applied there may be local pain and burning that disappears after several hours. Postoperative care includes regular cleansing of the peeled area and the application of an antibiotic ointment. Scabs may develop at the peel site. Healing is usually complete within two weeks, although the skin may remain red and sensitive for months.

An increase or decrease in normal skin pigmentation is the most common undesirable side effect of this procedure. An increase in pigment can be treated with bleaching medication or another peel if it doesn't resolve by itself. Loss of pigment, however, may be permanent. Scarring, usually in localized areas, can complicate chemical peels when the peeling agent (usually phenol) penetrates too deep into the skin.

DERMABRASION

This procedure, as it pertains to the treatment of acne scars, is discussed in detail in chapter 4. Dermabrasion has also been used to eliminate or modify scars from injuries, or from a bad case of chicken pox. The technique involves the use of a motor-driven, rapidly rotating abrading instrument such as a wire brush or a diamond burr. After the skin has been frozen with a spray-on refrigerant, the operator removes layers of the skin by abrading with varying degrees of pressure. In this manner shallow scars, irregularities, and discolorations can be removed. Dermabrasion is also used to lighten if not totally eliminate unwanted tattoos. In a tattoo removal, the skin is covered with a dressing after it has been dermabraded. The tattoo pigment then migrates to the surface, into the dressing. It may take several cycles of abrasion and healing to eliminate sufficient pigment for a cosmetic improvement to be readily apparent. Deeper dermabrasions, although more effective as far as pigment elimination is concerned, may heal with thick unattractive scars, a poor substitute for an unwanted tattoo (see chapter 13).

COLLAGEN INJECTIONS

The portion of the skin beneath the epidermis is made up of a large amount of fibrous protein called *collagen*. It is collagen that gives your skin its strength and suppleness. Alteration and loss of collagen occurs with aging, sun damage, and physical injuries that lead to scar formation.

In the past ten years, a form of purified collagen derived from cows has been used to correct scars and to modify exaggerated skin lines and furrows. Collagen is injected through a needle superficially into the area to be corrected. The immediate reaction is redness and swelling in the affected area, but in a few days this subsides and the injection sites blend in with the surrounding skin.

Prior to starting collagen treatments, a skin test with the bovine collagen is performed. About 3 percent of the population will test positive, indicating allergy to the protein. They are thus disqualified from treatment. Similarly, people with arthritis and other connective tissue diseases are not candidates for collagen because the foreign protein might aggravate their disease. Even after negative skin tests, some individuals will develop allergy after repeated collagen injections. This will likely manifest itself as a persistent bumpy swelling that may not resolve for many months. Another negative aspect of collagen therapy is its impermanence. Six to twelve months after treatment, the correction will start to fade away and further injections will be required to prevent a return to the pretreatment appearance.

Other materials used to fill in scars and other defects can include fibrin derived from the patient's blood, fat from the patient obtained by liposuction, and silicone. These materials have their advocates but they are not as widely used as collagen.

MOHS SURGERY

Although the Mohs surgical technique is not a cosmetic procedure, it has gained such popularity among dermatologists that it deserves mention. The Mohs method is used to remove skin cancers that have recurred after other forms of therapy, or to remove for the first time cancers that, by virtue of their type and location, have a high likelihood of recurring.

The Mohs method involves excising the tumor and immediately subjecting the quick-frozen tissue to careful microscopic examination to determine if the top, sides, and bottom of the specimen are free of tumor cells. If tumor cells are detected at any of the margins, then more tissue is immediately excised in the appropriate area of the wound. In some poorly defined skin cancers, multiple excisions are performed before the tumor is considered to be completely removed.

The wound left from the procedure may be closed with sutures or a skin graft or simply allowed to heal by itself. Sometimes a plastic surgeon will work with the Mohs surgeon in managing the wound after excision is complete. The Mohs method has a very high cure rate, although there is residual scarring. Nevertheless, it is not appropriate for most skin cancers that can be cured with simpler techniques, as described in chapter 11.

A BRIEF GLOSSARY

The information that follows provides some basic dermatological vocabulary intended to assist you in understanding a number of the words used in this guide. Although an effort has been made to use nonmedical equivalents throughout, accuracy sometimes demands the use of the exact medical term.

Acute condition A sudden, brief, and severe (as opposed to chronic) skin condition.

Alopecia Hair loss, baldness.

Axillary Of the armpit area of the body.

Bulla Blister.

Chronic condition A long-lasting or recurrent skin condition (and not as severe as an acute one).

Collagen The normal fibrous, connective tissue found in the skin and throughout the body.

Comedo Material obstructing a hair follicle opening, sometimes resulting in acne; a "blackhead." Also called *comedone.*

Corticosteroids A group of drugs based upon the structure of cortisone, a hormone produced by the adrenal glands.

Cyst A sac filled with liquid or semi-solid material.

Dermatitis An inflammation of the skin.

Dermis The portion of the skin under the epidermis, and made up largely of connective tissue.

Eczema A form of *dermatitis*; a specific skin condition sometimes called *atopic dermatitis* or *atopic eczema.*

Epidermis The paper-thin outer layer of the skin that is composed of multiple layers of cells.

Erosion A loss of epidermis; a superficial ulcer.

Erythema Redness of the skin.

Hemangioma An overdevelopment or tumor of the blood vessels.

Hyperpigmentation A condition of excess pigment or darkening of the skin.

Hypopigmentation A decrease in pigment, resulting in a lightening of the skin.

Keratin The complex protein material that makes up the hair and nails (and scales in some skin conditions). It is also a component of the epidermis.

Keratinization The process through which cells of the epidermis turn into keratin.

Melanin The brown skin pigment that imparts a color to the skin and develops with tanning.

Melanocyte Skin cell that produces melanin.

Miliaria A heat rash.

Mole A pigmented skin growth (a nevus).

Nevus A growth or spot on the skin, such as a birthmark or mole.

Nodule A solid, pea-sized (or larger) skin mass.

Papule A solid skin elevation smaller than a pea; a pimple.

Pruritus Itching of the skin, which can range from minor to severe.

Psychocutaneous Refers to the psychological aspects of skin function and disease.

Scale The thin, compacted cells of the epidermis that are shed from the skin.

Sebum The fatty material produced by the oil (sebaceous) glands.

Systemic Refers to the combined organs of the body, also to the internal administering of medications.

Topical medication Substances applied directly to the surface of the skin.

Tumor A swelling of the skin (not necessarily malignant).

Ulcer A loss of substance (skin layers) from the surface of the skin downward; an erosion.

Urticaria Hives, a condition characterized by the formation of wheals.

Verruca A wart.

Vesicle A small blister.

Xerosis Dryness of the skin.

SKIN PRODUCT RATINGS

INSECT REPELLENTS

The backbone of most insect repellents—the active ingredient that heads the list—is N,N-diethylmetatoluamide, nicknamed "deet." Generally regarded as the most effective repellent you can buy, deet defends against a broad array of biting pests.

The products surveyed ranged from about 5 percent deet to nearly 100 percent. They also have relatively small amounts of related compounds, or "isomers," that don't work as well as deet. Most repellents also contain inert ingredients like lotion bases or spray propellants.

Spraying insect repellent into the air offers no protection at all, and applying a repellent to one part of your body does not shield the rest of you. Clothing does afford some protection. But mosquitoes can bite right through T-shirts and other light-weight, tight-fitting garments. So experts recommend that you also apply repellent to clothing—inside and out, if you can.

On the other hand, insect repellents are potentially danger-ous if used continuously and excessively. Repellents should not be slathered onto naked limbs and torsos like sunscreens. Never spray them directly on the face. Instead, spray into the palm of one hand and use the fingertips of the other to apply the liquid on the face.

Recommendations

First consider products with smaller amounts of active ingredients. They're the ones least likely to cause skin reactions or other problems.

The Listings rank repellents by their percentage of active ingredients. Usually, the higher that percentage, the more hours of protection you can count on before you have to reach for the repellent again. Repellents that contain the chemical deet will likely work better and longer than those that rely on Rutgers 612—the products with the figure 612 in their name. Under all but the most extreme conditions, however, a product that's more than 50 or 55 percent deet is probably overkill.

Each form of repellent—spray, lotion, or stick—has its unique advantages. You may well get better coverage—and thus better protection—with an aerosol from the minimum-strength group than you do with a higher-strength lotion or stick—and less stickiness, too.

Listings

INSECT REPELLENTS

As published in *Consumer Reports*, July 1987.

Listed by percentage of total active ingredients. Except as noted, all use deet as their main active ingredient. All are effective against mosquitoes, ticks, chiggers, and fleas.

PRODUCT	TYPE	SIZE, OZ. OR FL. OZ.	ACTIVE INGREDIENTS/DEET [1]
Off!	Aerosol	6 [2]	15%/15%
Off! Pump Spray	Pump	3.5	15/15
Deep Woods Off!	Aerosol	6	25/20
Muskol Spray	Aerosol	6	25/25
Deep Woods Off! Pump Spray	Pump	3.5	25/20
Off! Towelettes	Towels	1.86	25/25
Cutter Original Spray Formula MMI	Aerosol	6 [2]	26/22
Cutter Evergreen Scent Spray Formula MMI	Aerosol	6 [2]	26/22
6/12 Plus [3]	Aerosol	7	30/ 5
Cutter Pump Spray Evergreen Scent	Pump	4	32/18
Cutter Stick Evergreen Scent	Stick	1	33/33
Cutter Stick	Stick	1	33/33
Deep Woods Off! Lotion Formula	Lotion	1	35/30
Deep Woods Off! Towelettes	Towels	1.86	38/32
Repel Spray	Aerosol	6	40/40
Muskol Ultra Maximum Strength Aerosol	Aerosol	6	40/40
Cutter Cream	Lotion	1	50/35
Cutter Cream Evergreen Scent	Lotion	1	50/35
Cutter Cream Single Use Packets	Lotion	0.76	50/35
Repel Spray Non-Aerosol Pump	Pump	4	55/55
Repel	Lotion	2	55/55
6/12 Plus Stick [3]	Stick	1	65/ 9

[1] Figures for deet include small amounts of related compounds (isomers).
[2] 12-oz. size also available.
[3] Major active ingredient is Rutgers 612 (see page 210).

211

SUNSCREENS

Most of the sun's effect on the skin is caused by a type of ultraviolet radiation called UVB. Another type, UVA, can cause photosensitive skin reactions in people taking certain drugs and may cause cataracts over time.

Most sunscreens are formulated to filter both UVA and UVB (the Ratings note the exceptions). As with melanin, the effectiveness of the sunscreen chemicals depends on how much is there to protect your skin.

The most obvious way to ensure that you have enough screening chemicals on your skin is to use a product with a high SPF. Compared with low-SPF products, such products have both a greater number of screening chemicals and more of each chemical. The U.S. Food and Drug Administration has set guidelines for determining SPFs. Our tests, both for this report and in the past, have shown that products do live up to their claimed SPF.

All the sunscreen in the world does no good if it's readily washed off. Most modern products make some claim of waterproofness or water resistance. The FDA has issued guidelines for substantiating such claims, so we decided to test a sampling of products to see if their claims for waterproofness or water resistance were well founded.

We applied sunscreen to people's backs, sat the subjects in a whirlpool, then "sunned" them under a high-powered Xenon-arc sunlamp. Sunscreens that claim to be waterproof had to maintain their SPF value through four twenty-minute "swims." Water-resistant sunscreens needed to stay strong through two twenty-minute swims. We tested the claims of about one-third of the products in the Ratings. All of them passed, so we assume the industry is generally abiding by FDA guidelines. Don't be lulled into feeling protected just because you buy a waterproof or water-resistant product. No matter how waterproof a sunscreen is, it still wipes off when you dry yourself with a towel after a swim or wipe the sweat from your brow during a tennis match. As some of the labels suggest, even waterproof products should be reapplied often.

Guide to the Ratings

Listed by types according to claimed water resistance. Tests of selected products showed that SPF and water-resistance claims are reliable.

1 *Product.* Regular sunscreen brands, cosmetics brands, and store brands.

2 *SPF.* The sun protection factor claimed on the label. You can find products in SPFs from 2 to 39; we tested mostly 15s.

3 *Form.* The traditional forms are lotions (**Lo**) and slightly thicker creams (**C**). Newer vehicles include gels (**G**); watery, alcohol-based liquids (**Li**); and aerosol sprays (**S**).

4 *Size.* Most products come in only one size of container.

5 *PABA-free.* While none of the products contain pure PABA (para-aminobenzoic acid), many contain PABA derivatives. If you're allergic to PABA, look here for products without such chemicals.

6 *Comments.* Look here for other aspects of these products that may affect your use. We've noted products with distinctive odors and those that feel oily or sticky.

Also note the products that can stain. We tested for staining on white cotton, polyester, cotton/polyester, nylon, and nylon/lycra fabrics. The products were applied, allowed to dry, and exposed to the equivalent of a day in the summer sun. We then washed the fabrics twice. All the sunscreens made nylon/lycra, a typical swimsuit material, pucker slightly. About half left yellow stains on some fabrics. We also tested the products on white fiberglass laminate such as what's often used in boats. Some stained it, caused it to swell, or dulled its finish slightly.

Ratings

SUNSCREENS

As published in *Consumer Reports*, June 1988.

1 PRODUCT	2 SPF	3 FORM	4 SIZE. OZ.	5 PABA-FREE	6 COMMENTS
WATERPROOF					
Sun Block (K Mart)	15	Lo	6	—	Medicinal odor.
Eckerd	15	Lo	6	—	—
Rite Aid	15	Lo	4	—	Stained nylon/lycra.
Burn-Off	16	Lo	4	√	Citrus odor, slightly oily, slightly sticky.
Alo Sun Fashion Tan	15	Lo	4	—	Sweet odor.
Super Shade	15	Lo	4	√	Stained nylon/lycra; sweet odor.
Hawaiian Tropic Baby Faces	25	Lo	4	√	Coconut odor.
Coppertone Water Babies	15	Lo	4	√	Sweet odor.
Hawaiian Tropic	15	Lo	4	—	Coconut odor; dulled shine on fiberglass.
Sea & Ski Block Out	15	S	4	—	Stained most fabrics, fiberglass; citrus odor.
Coppertone Vitamin E & Aloe	15	Lo	4	—	Stained cotton, polyester; sweet, spicy odor.
Sea & Ski Block Out Clear Lotion	15	Li	4	—	No UVA block; stained most fabrics, fiberglass; citrus odor.
Total Eclipse	20	S	4	—	No UVA block; stained most fabrics, fiberglass; sweet odor.
PreSun	15	Lo	4	—	Citrus odor; oily.
Sundown	15	Lo	4	—	Stained nylon/lycra; medicinal odor.
PreSun for Sensitive Skin	29	Lo	4	√	Oily.
Bain de Soleil Supreme	15	C	3⅛	—	Oily.
Li'l Gator	25	Lo	2	√	Stained nylon/lycra; slightly oily.
Lancôme Conquête du Soleil	15	Lo	4.2	—	Floral odor.
Bullfrog Amphibious Formula	18	G	1	—	No UVA block; stained polyester, nylon, nylon/lycra; chemical odor; oily and slightly sticky.

1 PRODUCT	2 SPF	3 FORM	4 SIZE, OZ.	5 PABA-FREE	6 COMMENTS
WATER-RESISTANT					
Avon Sun Seekers	15	Lo	4	—	Stained nylon/lycra; citrus odor.
Total Eclipse Oily & Acne Prone Skin	15	G	4	√	Stained nylon/lycra, fiberglass.
Ti-Screen	15+	Lo	4	√	Stained nylon/lycra; swelled fiberglass; oily.
Cancer Garde	33	Lo	4	—	Stained polyester, nylon, nylon/lycra.
Clinique Oil-Free	15	G	4	—	Stained nylon/lycra, fiberglass.
Ultima II	15	Lo	4	—	Stained cotton, nylon, nylon/lycra; spicy, medicinal odor; oily.
Clarins Ecran Total	18	Lo	1.7	√	Fleshtone; stained nylon, nylon/lycra; sweet citrus odor; oily and slightly sticky.
NO-CLAIM					
GNC Sun Bloc	15	Lo	4	—	No UVA block; coconut odor.
Nivea Sun	15	Lo	4	—	Herbal odor.
Almay Sun Block	15	Lo	3⅛	—	—
Doctors' Choice for Babies & Toddlers	23	Lo	4	—	Dulled fiberglass.
Doctors' Choice for Sensitive Skin	23	Lo	4	—	Dulled fiberglass.
Neutrogena	15	C	3	√	Fleshtone; oily.
Aramis Sun Series	15	Lo	3½	√	Stained nylon/lycra; swelled fiberglass.

LIPSTICKS

Do women buy a lipstick for its posh or panache? When we asked women readers what they looked for in a lipstick, they picked as important characteristics ease of application, moisturizing ability, color stability, staying power, and staying on the lips without feathering.

Can you get all those things in a single lipstick? No. A long-lasting lipstick may appear to change color over time. An extremely creamy lipstick may slide on easily, but will tend to feather and won't stay put. A waxy lipstick won't moisturize well.

The best you can do is decide which factor is most important to you and compromise on the others. If you like a very creamy lipstick, for example, you'll probably have to resign yourself to applying it more often.

Since women's priorities vary, we couldn't define any one set of qualities that make up a "good" lipstick. So the lipsticks in the Ratings are in order of price, from least to most expensive. Where possible, we evaluated three shades from each line, so our judgments would reflect characteristics of the line rather than of the individual colors. We chose a clear red, a pink, and an orange (which ranged in shade from light peach to deep coral).

In the lab, we tested to see which lipsticks would wash out of your clothes and which ones might melt in your purse. We noted which lipsticks come with a safety seal and which retract completely into the case. To characterize how the lipsticks looked, felt, went on, and came off, we turned to a professional makeup artist.

Recommendations

Nearly half our women readers use the same color of lipstick most of the time, our survey found. And half usually buy the same brand. That still leaves a lot of women who shop around. If you're one, the Ratings can be your guide.

Look in the Comments column for a lipstick with characteristics that appeal to you. We suggest starting with the drugstore lines. They're inexpensive, so you can experiment without investing much.

Certainly, if your present lipstick feels dry, feathers, wears off quickly, or is disappointing in some other regard, you should switch to another color or brand. The table below lists lipsticks that address specific problems.

If you're willing to pay department-store prices, you'll get a chance to try what you're buying. Don't apply the sample lipstick to your mouth. Instead, put a swipe of lipstick on your hand and hold it near your face.

You may find department-store clerks forthcoming about everything but price. So ask. If it's too high, don't hesitate to progress to the next glittering counter. Remember, all of them are selling pretty much the same inexpensive ingredients.

The colors you choose should match your skin tone. If you have yellowish or olive skin, peaches, corals, "warm" pinks, and orange-reds will look best. People whose skin has a blue undertone look good in clear reds and shades of pink.

Our makeup expert offers the following hints for applying lipstick:

- Use a brush. That's especially important for bright, opaque lipsticks, where precise control is especially important.
- Use a lip liner. Lining your lips will help define them and keep the color from feathering beyond the lip line. When you use pale, natural shades of lipstick, the liner should match your own lip color as closely as possible. With brighter shades, match the liner to the lipstick.
- Blot, reapply, and powder. This makes lipstick last for several hours. Blot and reapply your lipstick two or three times. Finish with a light dusting of face powder to set the lipstick.

Guide to the Ratings

Except as noted: All were moderate in the following qualities: gloss, creaminess, opacity, waxiness, ease of application, ease of removal, resistance to blotting, and tendency to stain lips.

1 *Brand and model.* Where possible, we tested a red, a pink, and an orange (shades of which ranged from light peach to coral) for each line. We list the manufacturer's color names in that order.

2 *Sealed.* A seal is important on less expensive lipsticks, which are kept out in the open in drugstores and supermarkets. All the drugstore lipsticks we tested except *Almay Moisturizing*, the *Coty* lines, and some samples of *L'Oréal* come sealed.

3 *Retractable.* Checked lipsticks retract completely into the case. With those that don't (usually cheaper models), it's easy to mangle the tip when you replace the top.

4 *Heat stable.* Our engineers heated lipsticks in an oven to see how well they withstood temperatures similar to those in a parked car on a hot summer's day. Those that stayed within the confines of their case earned a check.

5 *Fragrance.* Our trained "nose's" characterization of each lipstick's odor. Expensive lipsticks tend to be more strongly perfumed than cheaper models.

6 *Comments.* Our expert's evaluation of a variety of performance characteristics. As noted above, most lipsticks were moderately glossy, opaque, creamy, waxy, easy to apply, easy to remove, blot-resistant, and staining to the lips. Comments call out those that were notably high or low in those attributes. Look here for lipsticks with the qualities that are most important to you. Note that there's no reason to be brand-loyal. While some judgments are true for an entire line, most depend on color. So just because you like the red from one line, doesn't mean you'll like the pink.

RATINGS

LIPSTICKS

As published in *Consumer Reports*, February 1988.

1 BRAND AND MODEL	2 SEAL	3 RETRACTS FULLY	4 HEAT STABLE	5 FRAGRANCE	6 COMMENTS
Wet 'N' Wild 519, 527, 501	√	—	√	Waxy/greasy	Red was opaque and easy to apply; pink was glossy, easy to apply, nonstaining; coral was opaque, easy to remove, not blot-resistant, nonstaining.
Avon Coordinates (extra moist and shiny) *Different Apple, Porcelain Pink, Daring Peach*	—	√	—	Floral/sweet	Creamy, nonwaxy; red was opaque, easy to apply, staining; pink and coral were glossy, easy to remove, not blot-resistant, nonstaining.
Avon Coordinates (full color) *Rose Freeze, Pink Freeze, Cool Peach*	—	√	—	Faint floral/sweet	Glossy; red and pink were creamy, opaque, easy to apply, hard to remove; coral nonstaining.
Cutex Perfect Color (creams) *Classic Red, Soft Suede, Barely Buff*	√	—	√	Faint spicy/floral	Red was waxy, opaque, easy to apply, easy to remove, not blot-resistant, nonstaining; coral was opaque, easy to remove, not blot-resistant, nonstaining.
Cutex Perfect Color (frosts) *Brandy Wine, Satin Mauve, Fawn*	√	—	—	Faint fatty/spicy	Easy to apply, nonstaining; red was opaque, blot-resistant; pink was glossy, creamy, nonwaxy, blot-resistant; coral was glossy, sheer, creamy, nonwaxy, easy to remove.
Flame Glow Hours Longer *Cozumel Rose, Quiet Pink, Polished Coral*	√	—	—	Fatty/waxy	Waxy, opaque, easy to apply; red was easy to remove, not blot-resistant, nonstaining.
Cover Girl Luminesse 1 *Radiant Wine, Softpink Satin, Shimmering Shell*	√	—	—	Strong sweet	Glossy, creamy, nonwaxy, nonstaining; red was opaque, easy to apply, blot-resistant; coral was hard to apply, blot-resistant.
Revlon Natural Wonder Shiny Lips *Forever Red, Kiss Me Pink, Peaches 'N' Cream*	√	—	√	Sweet/soapy	Creamy, easy to remove, not blot-resistant; red was glossy, sheer, nonwaxy, easy to apply; pink was matte, easy to apply, nonstaining; coral was glossy, sheer, nonwaxy, nonstaining.

(continued)

219

1 BRAND AND MODEL	2 SEAL	3 RETRACTS FULLY	4 HEAT STABLE	5 FRAGRANCE	6 COMMENTS
Quencher Moisturizing Lustrous (with sunscreen) *All Wet Red, Poolside Pink, [coral not tested]*	✓	✓	✓	Sweet/spicy	Glossy, hard to remove; nonstaining; red was creamy.
Quencher Moisturizing Lustrous *Misty Plum (frost), Pink Meringue Frost, Frost Ice Tea*	✓	✓	✓	None	Glossy, creamy, opaque, easy to apply, hard to remove, nonstaining.
Maybelline Long Wearing *[red not tested], Iced Pink (frost), Rose Pink (cream) [coral not tested]*	✓	—	✓	Strong lanolin/floral	Creamy, blot-resistant, hard to remove; *Iced Pink* was sheer, glossy, hard to apply, nonwaxy; *Rose Pink* was opaque, easy to apply, staining.
Cover Girl Continuous Color *Red Royale, Spice Peach*	✓	—	✓	Strong sweet	Opaque, easy to apply; coral was creamy, easy to remove, non-staining, not blot-resistant; red was hard to remove, staining.
Maybelline Moisture Whip *Wine on Ice (frost), Sugar Plum (frost), Mocha ice*	✓	—	✓	Fatty/Waxy	Glossy, creamy, nonstaining; red was opaque, hard to remove, blot-resistant; pink was nonwaxy, hard to apply; coral was hard to remove.
Max Factor Maxi Soft Lustre Long Lasting *Red, [pink not tested], Coral*	✓	—	—	Strong tutti-frutti/bubble gum	Glossy, creamy, nonwaxy; red was easy to apply, hard to remove, staining; coral was opaque.
Max Factor Maxi-Moist Not Quite Lipstick *Streetsavvy Rose, Streetsmart Pink, First Flame*	✓	—	—	Strong tutti-frutti/bubble gum	Creamy, easy to remove, nonstaining; red was easy to apply, not blot-resistant; pink wasn't blot-resistant; coral was glossy, hard to apply.
Revlon Moon Drops Moisture Creme *Love That Red, Blazer Pink, Blasé Apricot*	✓	✓	✓	Soapy/spicy	Red is opaque, easy to apply, hard to remove, staining; both pink and coral were matte; pink was staining.
Almay Moisturizing *Dreamy Red, Perfect Pink, Melon Dares*	—	✓	✓	Faint waxy/greasy	Waxy; red and pink were sheer, hard to apply, and not blot-resistant; red was staining, pink wasn't; coral was hard to remove.
Coty Sheer to Stay *[red not tested], Starriest Pink, Sheerest Peach*	✓	—	—	Faint floral/sweet	Sheer, glossy; pink was hard to remove, coral was creamy, nonwaxy, easy to apply, nonstaining.

Product				Scent	Comments
Coty 24 *Coralline, Tea Rose, Persimmon*	—	✓	✓	Faint floral	Waxy, opaque, easy to apply, hard to remove, blot-resistant, staining; red and pink were glossy.
Revlon Moon Drops All Weather Lip Moisturizer *The Wine, Cool Pink, Dewy Melon* [1]	✓	—	—	Greasy/waxy	Glossy, creamy, sheer, nonwaxy, easy to remove, not blot-resistant, nonstaining; red and coral were easy to apply, pink was hard to apply.
Coty Silkstick *Perfect Red, Tender Pink, Fresh Roses*	—	✓	—	Sweet	Creamy; red was opaque, easy to apply, hard to remove; pink was easy to remove, nonstaining; coral was glossy, nonstaining.
Revlon Super Lustrous Creme *Fire & Ice, Pink in the Afternoon, California Sunshine*	✓	✓	✓	Faint sweet	Matte; red was opaque, easy to apply, hard to take off, stains; pink was creamy, nonwaxy, easy to apply and remove, not blot-resistant, nonstaining; coral sheer, was hard to apply, easy to take off, not blot-resistant, nonstaining.
L'Oréal L'Artiste Crème *Rouge, Pink Blush, Coral*	[2]	✓	✓	Fruity/leafy	Easy to apply; red was hard to remove, pink and coral were matte, noncreamy, opaque, waxy, easy to remove, not blot-resistant, nonstaining.
L'Oréal Crème Riche *Infrared, Pastel, Apricot*	—	✓	✓	Fruity	Matte, comes off when you blot; red was opaque, easy to apply, hard to remove; pink was noncreamy and hard to apply; coral was waxy, noncreamy, hard to apply.
Avon Ultra Wear *Persian Red, Jungle Melon, Island Coral*	—	✓	✓	Faint floral	Red was opaque, creamy, waxy, easy to apply, hard to remove, staining; pink was waxy; coral was glossy, sheer, creamy, hard to apply.
Francis Denney Moisture Silk Lip Color *Sultry Scarlet, Sweet Pink, Cool Melon*	—	✓	—	Faint floral	Opaque; red was glossy, easy to apply; coral was easy to apply; pink matte, easy to remove, nonstaining.
Clinique Re-Moisturizing *Zinnia, English Pink, Ripe Nectarine*	—	✓	✓	None	Red was opaque, waxy, easy to apply, hard to remove, staining; pink was glossy, sheer, creamy, easy to apply, easy to remove, not blot-resistant, nonstaining; coral was glossy.
Ultima II Super Luscious *Norell Red, Pink Vermeil, Coral Rose*	—	✓	✓	Sweet/waxy	Red was opaque, easy to apply, not blot-resistant, staining; pink was matte; pink and coral were sheer, creamy, hard to apply, easy to remove, not blot-resistant; coral was nonstaining.
Estée Lauder Re-Nutriv *Regal Red, Cinema Pink, Coral Melon*	—	✓	✓	Soapy/woody	Opaque, easy to put on; red was hard to remove, staining; pink was glossy, waxy, easy to remove, nonstaining; coral was waxy.
Lancôme Shining Lipcolor [3] *Peonie Sheer, Pink Cascade Sheer, Glory Sheer*	—	✓	✓	Strong rose	Glossy; nonstaining; red was sheer, creamy, nonwaxy, easy to apply, easy to remove; coral was easy to apply, blot-resistant; pink was creamy, blot-resistant.

(continued)

1 BRAND AND MODEL	2 SEAL	3 RETRACTS FULLY	4 HEAT STABLE	5 FRAGRANCE	6 COMMENTS
Ritz Perfect Finish Lipcolor *Clearly Red, Clearly Rose, Delicate Coral*	—	✓	—	Faint floral	Creamy, sheer; red was glossy, nonwaxy; pink was glossy, hard to apply, easy to remove, nonstaining; coral was hard to apply, easy to remove, not blot-resistant.
Elizabeth Arden Luxury Lacquer *Red, New Wave Pink, Nude*	—	✓	✓	Floral	Noncreamy, hard to remove, blot-resistant, nonstaining; red was easy to apply; pink was sheer; coral was opaque, easy to apply.
Estée Lauder Featherproof *Festive Red, Perfect Rose, Mandarin Melon*	—	✓	✓	Strong soapy/woody	Waxy; red was noncreamy, opaque, easy to apply, hard to remove, staining; pink was noncreamy matte; coral was glossy, opaque, easy to apply, nonstaining.
Germaine Monteil Creme Luxe *Vermilion, Fraise, Mango*	—	✓	✓	Sweet	Creamy, waxy; red was opaque, easy to apply, hard to remove, staining; pink was opaque, easy to apply; coral was matte.
Lancôme Hydrating Creme Lip Colour *Crimson, Pink Parallel, Fan Tango*	—	✓	✓	Strong rose	Creamy, nonstaining; red was opaque, hard to remove; pink was glossy, nonwaxy; coral was nonwaxy, opaque.
Princess Marcella Borghese Lumina Radiant Moisture *Radiccio, Nudo Pink, Viva Coral*	—	✓	—	Strong soap/sweet	Glossy; red was opaque, easy to apply, hard to remove; pink was creamy nonstaining; coral was creamy, opaque, easy to apply, easy to remove, nonstaining.
Chanel Rouge à Lèvres Super Hydrabase *Clear Red, Litchi French Pink, Cayenne Golden Coral*	—	✓	—	Strong rose	Opaque, easy to put on; red was glossy, creamy, waxy; pink was easy to remove, nonstaining; coral was waxy, hard to remove, staining; red and pink weren't blot-resistant, coral was.
Christian Dior *[red not tested]; Sheer Beryl, Vivid Orange*	—	✓	✓	Floral/berries	Creamy, nonwaxy; pink was easy to apply, easy to remove, nonstaining; coral was matte, sheer.
Yves Saint Laurent Fard à Lèvres *46, 30, 57*	—	✓	—	Strong herbal/tea rose	Creamy; red was opaque, easy to apply, blot-resistant; pink was hard to apply, easy to remove, nonstaining; coral was glossy, opaque, easy to apply.

1 Launderability better than for most brands tested.
2 Some samples came sealed; other did not.

HAIR MOUSSE

Mousse contains synthetic resins, which coat each hair with a thin, stiffening sheath. When the resins dry, they're stiff enough to hold a shape. Yet because each strand of hair is coated, you avoid the glued look, and the hair can still be combed.

The amount and the nature of the resins determines how much control a mousse allows. The more resin, the greater the control. And the more moisture-resistant the resins, the better a mousse will hold when the air is humid.

Other ingredients are there to condition hair, add moisture to it, or prevent static. Some of the ingredients make the mousse smell nice. There are also ingredients to force the liquid out of the can and others to make it foamy—to make it a mousse.

Many mousses contain alcohol, which is added to help dissolve the resins. But alcohol has a bad reputation in the world of hair, condemned as leaving hair looking too dry. So some mousse manufacturers have left alcohol out—and may use its absence as a selling point.

The Ratings reflect the hair-care factor our readers, in a survey, had identified as most important—how manageable the mousse makes your hair. All the mousses made hair more manageable. Those at the top of the Ratings did a better job than those at the bottom—but the differences were not dramatic.

Though any mousse should prove satisfactory at keeping your hair in place, you may choose one over another for any of the following reasons:

It adds body. Many of the mousses claim to do this. Our tests showed that three added more than moderate body.

It's cheaper. You can pay a lot less and still get a very serviceable mousse.

That difference in costs reflects two different marketing strategies. Cosmetic companies aim their products at the department-store set, while other brands are aimed at those who buy their cosmetics in the supermarket—and shop for the best price. You'll find budget brands throughout the Ratings.

It smells better to you. Some of the mousses we tested had a strong scent, others quite faint. But all had at least some noticeable fragrance. We characterize the fragrances in the Ratings.

It provides a sunscreen. Some people like the effect of sun-bleaching on their hair. If you don't, you may want to choose those which contain sunscreen chemicals. Or you may just decide to wear a hat.

It doesn't contain alcohol. Does alcohol really dry the hair? Our tests showed no correlation between lack of alcohol and good-feeling hair. There may be a correlation between the presence of alcohol and manageability, however: Few of the alcohol-free products made it to the top half of the Ratings.

Guide to the Ratings

Listed in order of manageability, based on judgments of a professional beautician who compared pairs of products on damp, shampooed hair. Differences between closely ranked products were judged not very significant.

1 *Product.* The control level is given in parentheses. Some lines offer more than one level of control; our tests showed that a brand's "extra" control usually outdid its "normal" control.

2 *Size.* To the nearest half-ounce.

3 *Added body.* Based on the beautician's judgment. Many products claim to add body—a feeling of thickness or density—to the hair. The beautician's judgments of bounce and fullness correlated closely with this judgment, so those factors are combined here. The same resins that add manageability also impart body, so the two assessments track fairly closely.

4 *Combing.* The beautician's judgment of how easy the hair was to comb out after the product had been applied and the hair blow-dried. The products that did best here let the comb slip easily through the hair, with no stickiness.

5 *Feel.* The beautician's judgment of whether the hair felt silky and pliable or stiff and harsh.

6 *Fragrance.* Our assessment. Sometimes the fragrance was very subtle. In other products, it was quite pronounced. Generally, the fragrance faded within half an hour.

Ratings

HAIR MOUSSE

● ◑ ○ ◐ ●

Better ←————————→ Worse

As published in *Consumer Reports*, October 1988.

1 PRODUCT	**2** SIZE, OZ.	**3** ADDED BODY	**4** COMBING	**5** FEEL	**6** FRAGRANCE	COMMENTS
Estée Lauder Swiss Styling	6	◑	◑	◑	Herbal/pine	A
Bryl-Creem Men's Grooming (Extra Control)	5	◑	○	◑	Citrus/pine	—
Breck Styling (Extra Style)	5	○	○	○	Spicy/floral	—
Pantene (Extra Firm Hold)	6	◑	○	○	Citrus/floral	A
Breck Styling (Light style)	5	○	◑	◑	Citrus/floral	—
L'Oréal Free Hold (Normal Control)	5	○	○	○	Minty/herbal/medicinal	—
Alberto European Styling Foam (Extra Control)	5½	○	○	○	Leafy/floral	—
White Rain (Extra Body)	5	○	○	○	Herbal	—
Avon Custom Control	4½	○	○	○	Citrus/floral	—
Jhirmack Nutri-Body (for fine, thin, limp hair)	5	○	○	○	Fruity	—
Jheri Redding Neutral (Firm Styling Formula)	6	○	○	○	Citrus/floral	—
Revlon Flex Body-Building (Extra Control)	5	○	◑	◑	Sweet/spicy	—
Wella Styling Mousse (for Fine/ Damaged Hair)	9	○	○	○	Floral	B
Vidal Sassoon for Men	6	○	○	◑	Spicy/floral	—

(continued)

225

1 PRODUCT	2 SIZE, OZ.	3 ADDED BODY	4 COMBING	5 FEEL	6 FRAGRANCE	COMMENTS
Alberto European Styling Foam (Normal Control)	5½	○	○	○	Leafy/floral	—
L'Oréal Free Hold (Extra Control)	5	○	○	◐	Herbal/medicinal	—
Wella Styling Mousse for Normal Hair	9	○	○	○	Floral	B
White Rain (Regular)	5	○	○	○	Herbal	—
Suave Styling Mousse (Normal Control)	5	○	○	○	Floral/herbal	—
Nexxus Nu-Set Mousse-Plus (Super Hold)	6	○	○	○	Medicinal	—
Pantene (Normal Hold)	6	◐	○	○	Citrus/floral	A
CVS Hair Styling Mousse (Extra Control)	5	○	○	○	Sweet/spicy	—
Alberto VO5 Thickening Hair Grooming Mousse for Men	5	○	◐	○	Spicy/medicinal	—
Créatif High Hold (Hold Factor 5L)	7	○	◐	◐	Spicy/floral/medicinal	A,B
Finesse (Extra Control)	5	◐	◐	○	Herbal/spicy	—
Clairol Condition (Extra Control)	6	◐	○	○	Leafy/floral	B
Finesse (Regular Control)	5	◐	○	○	Herbal/spicy	—
Dep Styling (Extra Control)	9	○	◐	○	Citrus/floral	B
Revlon Flex (Regular Control)	5	○	○	○	Spicy/floral/medicinal	—
Aqua Net (Extra Body)	5	○	○	◐	Sweet/spicy	B
L'Oréal Studio Line Sculpting Mousse	5	○	○	○	Fruity/spicy/medicinal	—
Clairol Condition (Normal Control)	6	○	○	○	Leafy/floral	B
Jhirmack Lite Frequent Use (Regular Hold)	5	○	○	○	Citrus/floral	—
Vidal Sassoon (Ultimate Hold for All Hair types)	8	◐	○	○	Almond	B
Tenax (Extra Control)	7	○	○	○	Spicy	B
Consort for Men (Thickening Formula)	8	○	○	○	Herbal	—
Gillette The Dry Look for Men (Regular)	5	◐	○	○	Herbal	—
Suave Styling Mousse Extra Control	5	◐	○	○	Floral/herbal	—
Vidal Sassoon (Full Body Formula for Fine Hair)	8	◐	○	○	Almond	B

Key to Comments

A–Contains sunscreen.
B–Does not contain alcohol.

SHAMPOOS

Despite the fancy ingredients and heavy-handed selling, shampoos can be relied on to do only one thing: They clean hair. Any other hoped-for effect is wishful thinking.

And all shampoos work in roughly the same way, using roughly the same tricks:

Cleaning agents. Surfactants are the working ingredients in all shampoos. They attract excess oil and dirt so that the offending compounds can be rinsed away along with the suds.

Soap is a surfactant. But it's not a good one for shampoo. Soap reacts with the minerals that make water hard, leaving a dulling film on the hair. (If you must use soap in a pinch, an acidic rinse such as lemon juice or vinegar will remove the film.)

Alternatives to soap, generally lumped together under the heading "detergent," don't leave a film. There are dozens of detergents, each with its own properties.

Baby shampoos generally contain mild surfactants. (Using mild surfactants and other relatively gentle ingredients helps prevent the shampoo from stinging if it gets in the eyes.)

Other surfactants are stronger. The ammonium lauryl sulfate and sodium lauryl sulfate touted by some shampoo makers are among the most common. They're especially effective at penetrating and removing oil and attacking residues of mousses, gels, and hair sprays.

In addition, there are surfactants that clean with little foam, and others that produce volumes of lather. Both varieties clean equally well.

Manufacturers generally use several surfactants in a single brand of shampoo. The number of possible combinations provides lots of room for claims of special formulas. It also provides the opportunity to formulate shampoos supposedly tailored for dry, normal, and oily hair.

According to a survey of *Consumer Reports* readers, more than half (62 percent) said they choose shampoo formulated for their "type" of hair. But whether you can tell the difference between one formula and another is doubtful.

227

Guide to the Ratings

Listed in order of estimated quality based on CU tests. All cleaned hair well.

1 *Product.* We tested best-selling national brands, store brands, and a couple of products sold only in hairstyling salons. Because shampoos made for specific hair types (normal, oily, etc.) are so common, we bought several brands in a selection of types.

2 *Overall quality.* Judgments were based on the behavior of the product during shampooing and the condition of the hair afterward. The best score was 96; the worst, 54. Differences of 7 points or more are significant.

3 *Price.* These are the average prices paid by CU shoppers in pharmacies, supermarkets, and, when necessary, hair salons in our area.

4 *Size.* With the exception of the concentrates (which are measured by weight), sizes are in fluid ounces. We tried to buy the shampoos in comparably sized containers, to keep cost comparisons fair.

5 *Cost.* Based on a total of 1½ teaspoons per shampoo (lathering twice). You may use less or more, but our costs serve as a convenient reference.

6 *Fragrance.* This is an important characteristic to many users. Descriptions are based on evaluation by CU chemists.

RATINGS

SHAMPOOS

As published in *Consumer Reports*, February 1989.

1 PRODUCT	2 OVERALL SCORE	3 PRICE	4 SIZE	5 COST PER USE	6 FRAGRANCE	COMMENTS
⊘ Pert Plus Extra Body For Fine Hair		$3.31	15 fl. oz.	6¢	Spicy/woody	A,B,C,D,E
⊘ Pert Plus Normal Hair		3.31	15	6	Spicy/woody	A,B,C,D,E
Nexxus Therappe		7.73	16	13	Coconut	K
Agree Extra Body Formula		3.23	15	6	Herbal	A,K
Ivory Fresh Scent Normal Hair		2.08	15	4	Sweet	—
Ivory Fresh Scent Oily Hair		2.08	15	4	Sweet	—
Ivory Fresh Scent Extra Body For Fine Hair		2.08	15	4	Sweet	—
Jhirmack E.F.A. Dry, Permed, Color Treated Hair		4.24	12	10	Citrus/tangerine	K
Pantene Extra Body For Fine Hair Thickening Formula		3.73	7	14	Herbal	—
Agree Regular Formula		3.23	15	6	Herbal	K
Perma Soft For Permed Hair Regular Formula		3.46	15	6	Floral/herbal	K
Halsa Swedish Botanical Formula Walnut Leaves		2.02	15	4	Herbal	—
Wella Balsam Conditioning For Extra Body		2.10	16	4	Citrus/floral	L
Revlon Flex Oily		2.15	15	4	Sweet/spicy	—

(continued)

⊘ This product was *check-rated*, judged high in quality and appreciably superior to other products tested.

229

PRODUCT	OVERALL SCORE	PRICE	SIZE	COST PER USE	FRAGRANCE	COMMENTS
Johnson's Baby Gentle Conditioning Formula		$3.92	15	7¢	Sweet/floral	—
Alberto VO5 Normal		1.35	15	2	Herbal/green leafy	—
Finesse Extra Body		3.45	15	6	Herbal	—
Silkience Self-Adjusting Extra Body		3.12	15	6	Medicinal/soapy	—
Redken Glypro-L For Fine/Normal Hair		10.58	16.9	17	Faint medicinal	K
CVS Balsam & Protein Treatment For Extra Body		1.49	16	3	Sweet/spicy	—
Wella Balsam Conditioning For Normal Hair		2.10	16	4	Citrus/floral	L
Helene Curtis Salon Selectives Level 7 Deep For Normal To Oily Hair		2.38	15	4	Fruity	K
Suave Full Body Normal/Dry Hair		1.56	16	3	Woody/spicy	—
Silkience Self-Adjusting Regular		3.12	15	6	Medicinal/soapy	—
CVS Balsam & Protein Treatment For Normal To Dry Hair		1.49	16	3	Sweet/spicy	L
Revlon Flex Normal To Dry		2.15	15	4	Sweet/spicy	—
Avon Natural Brilliance		2.49	16 fl. oz.	4	Faint floral	—
Suave Moisturizing Regular		1.56	16	3	Woody/spicy	—
Alberto VO5 Extra Body		1.35	15	2	Herbal/green leafy	—
White Rain Regular		1.65	18	2	Floral/faint herbal	—

Product					
Clairol Condition Revitalizing Formula For Normal Hair		1.99	15	4	Sweet/spicy	—
K Mart Balsam Treatment Normal To Dry Hair		1.28	16	2	Sweet/spicy/herbal	—
Breck Balanced Cleaning & Conditioning For Normal Hair		1.63	15	3	Herbal/spicy	—
Head & Shoulders Normal To Dry [bottle]		4.20	15	8	Sweet/slightly spicy	—
Revlon Flex Extra Body		2.15	15	4	Sweet/spicy	—
Breck Extra Conditioning For Dry, Damaged Or Color Treated Hair		1.63	15	3	Herbal/spicy	—
Suave Extra Gentle Extra Body		1.56	16	3	Woody/spicy	—
Perma Soft For Permed Hair Extra Body Formula For Fine/Limp Hair		3.46	15	6	Floral/herbal	K
Clairol Condition Extra Body Formula For Fine Limp Hair		1.99	15	4	Sweet/spicy	—
Halsa Swedish Botanical Formula Chamomile		2.02	15	4	Herbal	—
Affinity		3.24	15	6	Floral	K
Pantene For Normal Hair Daily Use Formula		3.73	7	14	Floral/hyacinth	—
Truly Fine Balsam and Protein Treatment For Normal To Dry Hair (Safeway)		1.47	15	3	Spicy	—
Finesse Regular		3.66	15	7	Herbal	—
Vidal Sassoon Advanced Salon Formula For Normal Hair		3.68	12	8	Marzipan/almond	—
Ivory Dishwashing Liquid		1.54	22	2	Sweet	L
Jhirmack Geláve Gel Normal Hair		4.24	12	10	Floral/herbal	K
White Rain Extra Body		1.65	18	2	Floral/faint herbal	—

(continued)

231

1 PRODUCT	2 OVERALL SCORE 0–100	3 PRICE	4 SIZE	5 COST PER USE	6 FRAGRANCE	COMMENTS
Johnson's Baby		3.59	15	6	Sweet/floral	—
Avon Natural Brilliance For Dry/Damaged Hair		2.49	16	4	Faint floral	—
Kroger Extra Balsam & Protein Treatment Normal To Dry Hair		1.37	15	2	Sweet/spicy/herbal	—
Vidal Sassoon Advanced Extra Body For Fine or Limp Hair		3.68	12	8	Marzipan/almond	—
Nexxus Assure		6.92	16	12	Citrus	H,K
Helene Curtis Salon Selectives Level 5 Regular For Normal Hair		2.38	15	4	Fruity	—
Prell Normal To Dry Hair [bottle]		3.42	15	6	Herbal/spicy	K
Fabergé Organics With Extra Body Ingredients		1.68	15	3	Herbal	G
Fabergé Organics		1.68	15	3	Herbal	G
Redken Classic Amino Pon For Chemically Treated Hair		10.31	16.9	17	Fruity	F,H,I,K
Prell Concentrate Normal To Dry Hair [tube]		3.30	7 ☐	15	Herbal/spicy	F,H,I,J,K
Head & Shoulders Concentrate Normal To Dry [tube]		3.53	5.5 ☐	20	Sweet/slightly spicy	F,H,I,J,K

☐ Ounces, not fluid ounces.

Key to Comments

A–More generous lathering than most.
B–Faster, richer, more emollient, and longer-lasting lather than most.
C–Easier to rinse out than most.
D–Allowed easier wet combing than most.
E–Left dry hair silkier and easier to comb than most.
F–Lathered less than most.
G–Lathered slower than most.
H–Lathering was slower and suds were coarser than most.
I–Lather faded faster than most.
J–More difficult to rinse out than most.
K–Thicker than most tested shampoos.
L–Thinner than most tested shampoos.

INDEX

Abrasive therapy, 41
Accutane (isotretinoin), 34, 45, 46, 47, 49, 73, 150
Acne, 2, 36–50, 62, 79, 94
    causes of, 36–40
    infantile, 176
    stages of, 47
    treatment of, 40–50, 78, 80
Acne rosacea, 191–92, 199–200
Acrodermatitis enteropathica, 77–78
Acute glomerulonephritis, 181
Acyclovir, 117, 118, 128, 129
Adrenal glands, 28, 32, 37, 93, 172
Aging of skin, 8, 146, 149, 159
AIDS (acquired immune deficiency syndrome), 112, 129, 132–33
Albinism, 171
Allergens, 60
Allergic contact dermatitis, 22, 26, 27, 28, 52–67, 91, 148
    causes of, 59–61
Allergic reactions, 18–19, 30, 106, 110–11, 138–39, 186, 195
Allergies, 13, 26, 51–70, 103, 169
    in atopic dermatitis, 20–21, 22
    delayed, 52
Aloe vera, 145

Alopecia areata, 89–90
Ammonia, 178
Amobarbital, 64
Amphotericin B, 101, 122, 179
Anaphylaxis, 138
Androgens, 37–38, 86, 87, 93–94
Anemia, 74, 85–86, 102, 167
Anesthetic creams, 128, 138
Anesthetics, 30, 84, 106, 108
    see also "-caine" anesthetics
Angioneurotic edema, 70
Anti-androgens, 49–50, 88
Antibacterial ointment, 138
Antibiotic ointments, 29, 98, 100, 114, 117, 178, 179, 181, 202
Antibiotics, 16, 21, 23–24, 62, 89, 100, 106, 137
    oral, 114, 115, 162
    systemic, 28, 181
    in treatment of acne, 43–45, 47
    in treatment of dermatitis, 25–26
    in treatment of infectious diseases, 124, 126, 186
    in wet dressings, 23–24
Antibodies, 52, 65, 109
Antifungal medications, 101, 102, 107, 109–10, 111, 121, 123, 133, 178, 179

Antihistamines, 29, 30, 61, 62, 63, 138, 142
  oral, 30, 196
  in treatment of drug reactions, 65, 69
Anti-itch medications, 20, 30, 61–62, 142, 188
Antiseptics, 62
Aphthous stomatitis, 108
Apocrine glands, 10, 11
Arsenic, 151, 167
Arthritis, 32, 123, 124, 167, 203
Aspirin, 29, 64, 67, 106, 145, 185, 189
Asthma, 18, 167
Athlete's foot, 101, 120
Atopic dermatitis (eczema), 2, 18–22, 27, 62, 102, 84–85, 133, 192
Autoallergic (autoimmune) illness, 108, 109, 172
Autoimmune response, 90
Autonomic nervous system, 190
Autosensitization, 18

Bacitracin, 26, 179, 181
Bacteria, 75, 98, 113–14, 161–62
  and acne, 36, 38, 41, 43
Bacterial infections, 21, 98, 100, 113–16, 185, 186
  and diaper rash, 178, 179
  impetigo, 180–81
  prevention of, 117, 118
Baldness (alopecia), 16, 85, 86–91
Barbiturates, 63, 64
Basal cell carcinoma, 150–52
Bathing, 15, 22–23, 29
Bees, 52, 137–38, 167
Benign skin growths, 156–63
Benzoyl peroxide, 40, 41, 45, 47
Berloque dermatitis, 166
Beta carotene, 72, 73
Birth control and Accutane, 46
Birth control pills, 45, 64, 83, 122
  and pigmentation, 165–66, 167
Birth defects, 46, 150

Birthmarks, 181–84, 199
Bites, 134–42, 180
"Black, hairy tongue," 109–10
Blackheads, 36, 40, 46–47
Blacks, 151, 157, 165, 168, 182
Bleaching creams, 168
Blisters, 8, 13, 109, 116
  with excessive sweating, 193–94
  fever, 21, 108, 111, 116, 180
  in heat rash, 176–77
  with herpes, 117, 128
  with poison ivy, 53, 54
Blood tests, 131, 132
Blood vessels, 9, 12, 13, 17, 77, 190
  birthmarks composed of, 181, 183
  permanently dilated, 27
  supersensitive, 191, 192
Body odor, 10–11
Boils, 21, 47, 114–15
Bowen's disease, 153
Bromhidrosis, 10–11
Bromides, 63
Burning mouth syndrome, 105–6

"-caine" anesthetics, 57, 61, 62, 145, 148
Calamine lotion, 24, 54
Cancer, 129, 194
  see also Skin cancer
Candida albicans (thrush), 43, 100, 106–7, 111, 121–22, 178
Candidiasis, 132
Canker sores (aphthae), 107–8, 112
Carbohydrates, 78–79
Carotenemia, 73
Cauterization, 107, 108
Chancre, 131
Chemical additives, 67–68
Chemical depilatories, 94, 95
Chemicals, 14, 59, 110, 130, 170
Chemotherapy, 34, 85, 151, 161, 167
Cherry spot, 161
Chicken pox, 31, 117–18, 132, 185–86

Children, 196
  dermatology for, 175–89
Chloasma, 166
Chronic skin disease, 2, 31, 94
Circulation, 17, 102
Club hairs, 82–83
Clubbing, 102
Cold, allergies to, 69
Cold sores, 21, 111, 116
Collagen, 8, 80, 203
Comedones. See Whiteheads (come-
  dones)
Compresses, 23–24, 29, 54, 117,
  118, 162
Congenital moles, 182
Congenital syphilis, 131
Connective tissue, 8, 9, 27, 28
Corticosteroid ointments, 16, 29,
  55, 190–91, 195–96
Corticosteroids, 33, 34, 70, 90, 102,
  109, 137, 138, 142, 183, 184
  with acne, 45, 47
  with dermatitis, 25, 26–28
  with drug reactions, 65
  with sunburn, 145
  systemic, 28, 55–56, 57
  use with children, 179, 180
Cortisone, 94
Cosmetic allergy, 58–59
Cosmetic procedures, dermatologi-
  cal, 198–204
Cosmetic surgery, 49, 198–201
Cosmetics, 41, 80, 103, 173–74
Coxsackie virus, 187
"Crabs." See Pubic lice
Cradle cap, 179
Cross-sensitization, 57–58, 148
Crude coal tar, 33
Cryosurgery (freezing), 130, 152,
  157
Cystic acne, 36, 45, 46
Cysts, 161–62, 200

Dandruff, 16–17, 79, 84, 139
Dehydration, 11–12
Dermabrasion, 48–49, 169, 202

Dermal-epidermal junction, 8
Dermatitis, 13–30, 170
  treatment of, 22–29
Dermatofibromas, 162–63
Dermatologists, 1–3, 30, 152
Dermatopathologists, 2
Dermis, 6, 8, 12, 48
Dermographism, 69
Desensitization, 18–19, 54, 56, 69,
  139
Diabetes, 66, 122, 194
Diaper rash, 177–79
Diet, 16, 20, 72
  and acne, 39–40
  balanced, 71, 76, 77, 78, 80
  elimination, 68–69
Diet diary, 68, 69
Diet therapy, 79, 191
Diethylmetatoluamide (deet), 135,
  137, 209
Diets, 78–79, 84
Discoloration of skin, 17, 78
Disease, 69, 83–84, 102
  of nails, 100–3
Dressings, 29
Drug reactions, 62–65, 66
Dry skin, 20, 194
Dry skin dermatitis, 15–16, 30
Dyshidrosis, 193–94
Dysplastic nevus syndrome, 159

Eccrine glands, 10, 11, 12
Eczema, 2, 18–22, 27, 62, 84–85,
  102, 133, 192
Electrodesiccation, 152, 160, 192,
  200
Electrolysis, 94, 95
Electrosurgery, 130, 157, 160, 161,
  192, 199–200
Emotional factors
  in acne, 38–39
  in atopic dermatitis, 21–22
  in hair loss, 84
  in herpes, 117
  in hives, 69–70
  in shingles, 118

Emotional factors (*cont'd*)
and skin disorders, 12, 190–97
Emulsions, 24–25, 30
Epidermal cells, 6, 8, 9, 32, 41, 109, 173
Epidermal nevi, 182
Epidermis, 5–6, 8, 48, 72, 95, 144
Epidermoid cysts, 161–62
Epinephrine, 138
Erysipelas, 115–16
Erythema multiforme, 108–9
Erythromycin, 21, 44, 45, 114, 181, 186
Erythroplakia, 107
Estrogen, 45, 87, 165
Etretinate, 34–35, 73
Eyes, 72–73, 171, 172

Facial hair, 93, 94
Fats, 78–79
Fetus, 35, 131, 185
Fever blisters, 21, 108, 111, 116, 180
Fevers, 184–89
Fifth disease (erythema infectiosum), 187
"Fixed" drug reaction, 63–64
Fleas, 135
Flies, 137
Folliculitis, 114
Food allergies, 20, 67–69, 108
Food and Drug Administration (FDA), 88, 150, 212
Formaldehyde, 103, 119
Formication, 196–97
Freckles, 157, 168
Fungal infections, 121–23, 132, 171, 195
and diaper rash, 178, 179
of nails, 100–3
Fungus, 120

Gamma rays, 143
Genetic factors
in acne, 37
in aging of skin, 159
in allergies, 51
in atopic dermatitis, 20
in baldness, 86
in pigmentation, 165
in seborrheic dermatitis of infancy, 179
Genital areas, 10, 27, 109, 117, 195
Genital herpes simplex, 128–29
"Geographic" tongue, 110
German measles (rubella), 185
Gnats, 137
Goeckerman regimen, 33, 34
Gold, 56, 63
Gold salts, 167
Gonorrhea, 126
Griseofulvin, 101, 121

Hair, 8–10, 81–95
excess, 93–95
growth of, 82–83
Hair care, 92–93
Hair cycle, 82, 83, 84
Hair damage, 91–92
Hair dye, 91, 92–93, 148
allergy to, 57–58
Hair follicles, 8–9, 36, 48, 84, 93, 95
infections of, 114–15
Hair implants, 88–89
Hair loss, 45, 77, 79, 91
reasons for, 83–94
treatment of, 84–86
Hair mousse Ratings, 223–25, *226–26*
Hair procedures, cosmetic, 91–93
Hair pulling, 196
Hair transplant, 88–89
Hairstyling, 90–91, 92
Hand, foot, and mouth disease, 187
Hangnails, 98
Heat rash (miliaria), 176–77
Heliotherapy, 42
Hemangiomas, 183
Hereditary defects, 13, 31
see also Genetic factors
Herpes simplex, 111, 116–17, 132

Herpes simplex virus, 21, 108
Herpes zoster (shingles), 116–17, 132, 186
Histamine, 67
Histiocytomas, 162–63
Hives. *See* Urticaria (hives)
Hormonal factors in acne, 37–38
Hormones, 45, 83, 84, 86, 93–94, 165
Hydrocortisone, 26, 28
Hydroquinone, 168, 170
Hygiene, 40, 115, 134
  poor, 140, 195
Hyperhidrosis, 12, 192–94
Hyperpigmentation, 165–68
Hyperthermia, 12
Hypertrichosis, 87, 93–94
Hypoallergenic cosmetics, 59
Hypopigmentation, 170–74

Ibuprofen, 145
Immune response, 21, 109, 186
Immune system, 51, 58, 172, 180
Impetigo, 21, 111, 176, 180–81
Infants, 106, 176
  eczema, 19
  herpes infection, 129
  seborrheic dermatitis, 179–80
  skin, 175–76, 180
Infections, 13, 69, 85, 113–26
  and acne, 38
  with atopic dermatitis, 21
  causing hypopigmentation, 171
  in infants, 175–76, 180
  of nails, 100–2
  and sexually transmitted diseases, 113–33
  see also Bacterial infections; Fungal infections; Viral infections
Infectious diseases, 123–26
Infectious mononucleosis, 112, 187–88
Infestations, 134, 140, 196–97
Inflammation, 165
Insect bites. *See* Bites
Insect repellents, 135, 137

Ratings of, 209–10, *211*
Intertrigo, 177–78
Iodine, 62, 63
Iron deficiency, 77, 85–86, 102
Irritations, 13, 18, 106
Itching (pruritus), 20, 27, 194–96
  in eczema, 19–20
  relief of, 28–29, 30, 55, 70
Itch-scratch cycle, 19, 195–96

Jellyfish, 142
Jock itch, 120

Kaposi's sarcoma, 132–33
Kawasaki disease, 188–89
Keloids, 48
Keratin, 7, 10, 14, 96
Keratinization, 6–7, 9, 10, 32, 36, 72
Keratoses, 159–61, 200
Keratosis pilaris, 20
Ketoconazole, 101, 121, 122
Kidney disease, 103, 194
Koplik spots, 184
Kwashiorkor, 78

Lasers, 169, 183, 184, 198–99
Laxatives, 64
Lentigines, 157
Leprosy, 171
Leukemia, 85
Leukoplakia, 107
Lice, 139–40
Lichen planus, 107
Lidocaine, 106, 108, 128
Light rays, 143, 147
  and pigmentation, 164, 165
  see also Ultraviolet light
Lindane, 127, 139–40, 141
Liposuction, 200–1, 203
Lips, 105–12
  contagious conditions affecting, 111–12
  problems of, 110–12
Lipstick Ratings, 216–18, *219–22*
"Liver" spots, 157, 200

Lotions, 24–25, 29, 30
Lyme disease, 123–25, 137
Lymph glands, 185, 188–89
Lymphocytes (white blood cells), 52, 65

Malaria, 67, 167
Male pattern baldness, 9, 16, 86–89
Malignant melanoma, 150, 153–55, 157, 159, 182
Measles (rubeola), 116, 184–85
Medication burns, 106
Medications, 34–35, 103, 117, 194
    allergic reactions to, 52, 61–65, 67
    and hair loss, 85
    hyperpigmentation from, 167–68
    sunlight in conjunction with, 65–66
    systemic, 28–29
Melanin, 7–8, 65, 151, 156, 164, 171, 173, 212
    absence of, 171–72
    in tanning, 146
Melanocyte(s), 7–8, 146, 156, 172–73
    birthmarks derived from, 182
    and pigmentation, 164
Melasma, 165–66, 167, 168
Menstruation, 85, 94, 117
Mercury, 56, 62, 168, 169
Metals, allergy to, 56
Methotrexate, 34, 35
Miconazole, 101, 121, 122, 179
Milia, 176
Miliaria, 176–77
Minerals, 71, 77–78, 80
Minoxidil, 87–88, 90, 94
Moisturizers, 15–16, 20, 41
Moles, 153, 154, 156–59, 199
    congenital, 158–59, 182
    removal of, 157–58
Molluscum contagiosum, 129–30, 132
Mongolian spot, 182
Mosquitoes, 137

Mouth, 105–12
Mucocutaneous lymph node syndrome, 188–89

Nail biting, 98–99, 104
Nail injuries, 98, 99
Nailectomy, 100
Nails, 32, 96–104, 120, 121
    brittle, 97
    care of, 103–4
    cuticle, 97, 98–99, 103
    diseases of, 100–3
    ingrown, 99–100
    lunula, 97
    matrix, 96, 97, 99
    split, 97
    spots, lines, furrows, 99
    and subtle symptoms, 102–3
Neomycin, 26, 62, 179
Nephritis, 181
Neuralgia, postherpetic, 118
Neuritis, 118
Neurodermatitis, 195
Nevi
    dysplastic, 159
    epidermal, 182
Nevus flammeus (port-wine stain), 183, 199
Niacin, 75–76
Nutrition, 71–80
Nutritional deficiency, 97, 105–6
Nystatin, 101, 107, 111, 122, 179

Obesity, 17, 122
Oil (skin), 10, 37
Oil glands, 46, 48
Onycholysis, 103–4
Over-the-counter medications, 30, 54–55, 121, 145, 168
    acne, 40, 41, 47
    allergies to, 61–62

Papillae, 9
Papules. See Pimples
Para-aminobenzoic acid (PABA), 57–58, 65, 111, 148, 213
Paronychia, 100–1

Patch testing, 60–61
Pediatric skin problems, 175–89
Peeling, 40, 41
Pellagra, 75–76
Pemphigus, 109
Penicillin, 21, 26, 62, 114, 116, 124, 126, 186
  allergic reactions to, 62, 63, 67
  in treatment of syphilis, 130, 131, 132
Petroleum jelly (petrolatum), 25, 30
Pharmaceutical industry, 24, 27
Phenacetin, 64
Phenol, 170, 201–2
Photosensitive skin reactions, 212
Phototherapy, 33–34
Phototoxic rash, 166–67
Phrynoderma, 72
Phytophotodermatitis, 166
Piebaldism, 171
Pigment loss, 202
Pigmentation, 8, 45, 48, 164–74, 202
Pigmented skin growths, 153–54
Pimples, 36, 40, 176, 180
Pityriasis alba, 170
Pityriasis rosea, 188
Plantar warts, 119
Plastic surgery, 198
Poison ivy (Rhus radicans), 53–56
Polymorphous light eruptions, 66, 67
Postscabies syndrome, 141–42
Pregnancy, 35, 43, 46, 83, 150, 165, 185
  and genital herpes, 129
  and pigmentation, 165–66
  and syphilis, 131
Prickly heat, 177
Protein, 76, 78–79, 84
Psoralen, 33, 173
Psoriasis, 2, 31–35, 62, 84–85, 102, 192, 195
  diet therapy for, 79
  treatment of, 32–35, 173
Psychosomatic disorders, 12

acne as, 38–39
  see also Emotional factors
Psychotherapy, 21
Pubic lice, 127–28, 139
Purpura, 17, 63
Pustules, 36, 46
PUVA, 33–34

Quinidine, 63
Quinine, 63

Radiation, 146–47, 151, 165
Radiation treatment, 151, 183, 184
Radiotherapy, 152
Rashes, 52–53, 170
  in children, 184–89
  in drug reactions, 63
  of eczema, 19
  emotionally triggered, 191
  in erysipelas, 116
  in fungal infections, 122
  in irritant contact dermatitis, 14
  in Lyme disease, 123–24
  phototoxic, 166
  in poison ivy, 53
  in scabies, 140–41, 142
  seborrheic, 16
  in shingles, 118
  in sun allergy, 65
  from topical medications, 41
Ratings, skin products (Consumer Reports), 3, 209–32
Repigmentation, 172–73
Respiratory infections, 112
Retin-A. See Tretinoin
Retinoids, 73–74, 85, 107
Riboflavin, 76
Rickets, 75
Rickettsialpox, 125
Ringworm, 120–21, 132
Rocky Mountain spotted fever, 125–26, 137
Roseola infantum, 186–87
Rubber allergy, 57

Salabrasion, 169–70
Salicylates, 67

Salicylic acid, 16, 40, 47, 119, 179
Scabies, 139, 140–42
Scalp, 16, 120, 121
Scarlet fever, 186
Scarring, 45, 47, 50, 202, 204
Scars, 48–49, 183, 184, 202
Sclerotherapy, 18, 200
Scraping (treatment), 130, 160
Scratching, 19, 29, 195–96
Scurvy, 77
Sebaceous cysts, 161–62
Sebaceous glands, 8, 10, 36, 50, 79, 80
Seborrheic dermatitis, 16–17, 27, 76, 79, 178, 192
    in AIDS patients, 133
    and hair loss, 84
    in infancy, 179–80
Seborrheic keratoses, 157, 159–60
Sebum, 10, 36, 37, 38, 41, 46
Selenium sulfide, 16, 123
Sensitivity to sun, 65–67
Sensitization, 26, 53, 57
Sexually transmitted diseases (STDs), 126–33
Shampoo(s), 16, 92, 179–80
    medicated, 84, 139–40
    Ratings of, 227–28, 229–32
Shaving, 94, 114
Shingles (herpes zoster), 116–17, 132, 186
Side effects, 34–35, 67, 80, 184, 193
    of acne medications, 46
    of antibiotics, 43–44, 102
    of corticosteroids, 27, 28, 32–33, 45, 90
    of dermabrasion, 48
    with hair transplant, 89
    of hormones, 45
    of Retin-A, 149
Silicone, 203
Silver, 56, 103
Sitz baths, 128
Skin, 5–12
    cumulative damage to, 146–50
    structure of, 5–8

Skin cancer, 34, 94, 167, 171, 173
    benign skin growths and, 157–58, 159, 160–61, 162
    sun and, 150–55
    surgery in treatment of, 200, 203–4
Skin diseases
    infectiousness of, 113
Skin disorders, 198–99
    emotions and, 190–97
Skin dyes, 173–74
Skin peels, 201–2
Skin product Ratings. See Ratings
Skin testing, 20, 68, 69
Skin types, 144
Smallpox, 21
Soap, 14, 15, 16, 40, 47, 227
Solar keratoses, 152–53, 160–61
Sores (mouth), 107–9
Spider angiomas, 200
Spiders, 136–37
Spiny cells, 7
Squamous cell carcinoma, 150, 152–53, 160
Staphylococcus bacteria, 47, 100, 114–15, 126, 180
Stasis dermatitis, 17, 18
Steroids. See Corticosteroids
Stevens-Johnson syndrome, 108–9
Stings, 134–42
Strawberry mark (capillary hemangioma), 183
Streptococcus bacteria, 116, 180, 181, 186
Streptomycin, 26, 63
Stress, 38, 108, 190
Stretch marks, 27
Sulfa drugs, 26, 57, 63, 148
Sulfonamides, 62, 66
Sulfur, 16, 40, 47, 180
Sun allergy, 65–67, 144, 148
Sun blisters, 116
Sun damage (skin), 8, 80, 111, 159, 160, 161, 201
Sun protection factor (SPF), 148–49, 212
Sunburn, 31, 144–45, 146, 148, 172

sensitivity to, 44
Sunburst veins, 200
Sunlight
  allergic reactions to, 52
  and pigmentation, 170
  and skin cancer, 143–55
  therapeutic value of, 41–42
  vitamin D from, 74–75
  see also Ultraviolet light
Sunscreens, 65, 66–67, 146, 147–50
  Ratings of, 212–13, 214–15
Surfactants, 227
Surgery, 84, 88–89, 199
Surgical treatment
  of acne, 46–47
  of birthmarks, 183–84
  of moles, 159
  of skin cancer, 151–52, 153, 155
  of varicose veins, 18
  of warts, 119
Sweat glands, 8, 10–12, 176, 190,
  192–94
Sweating, excessive (hyperhidrosis),
  12, 192–94
Swelling (edema), 13, 17
Syphilis, 126, 130–32, 167

Tanning, 42, 144, 146, 165
Tar ointments, 16, 33
Tattoos, 169–70, 199, 202
Telogen effluvium, 83
Tetracycline, 43–44, 45, 64, 103,
  108, 122, 124, 126, 192
  reactions to, 66
Thamine (vitamin B_1), 137
Thickening of skin, 13, 17, 19
Thinning of skin, 27, 32
Thrombophlebitis, 17
Thyroid disease, 103, 194
Thyroid gland, 85, 172
Thyroid pills, 85
Ticks, 124–25, 137
Tinea versicolor, 122–23, 171
Tongue, 105, 109–10
Topical antibiotics, 25–26, 27, 44–
  45, 47
  see also Antibiotic ointments

Topical medications, 17, 26–28,
  32–33, 40–41, 179
Toxic shock syndrome, 126
Traction baldness, 90–91
Tranquilizers, 29, 63, 66, 191, 193,
  196
Treatment of skin disorders. See in-
  dividual disorders
Trench mouth, 111–12
Tretinoin (Retin-A), 40, 41, 45, 47,
  73, 80, 149–50, 168
Trichloroacetic acid, 119, 201–2
Tumors, benign, 119

Ulcers, 17, 107–9
Ultraviolet light, 8, 65
  therapy from, 33–34, 41–42, 173
Ultraviolet rays, 143–44, 147, 148,
  164
  and pigmentation, 164, 165
  UVA and UVB waves, 33–34,
  144, 146, 148, 212
Urea, 15–16
Urticaria (hives), 52, 63, 65, 67–70,
  138, 192

Vaccines, 184, 185, 186
Vaginal infection, 43, 45, 122
Varicose veins, 17, 18
Varicosities, 200
Vellus hairs, 9
Venereal warts, 130
Viral hepatitis, 112
Viral infections, 116–20, 132
Vitamin A (retinol), 47, 72–74, 79,
  80, 85, 107
Vitamin B complex, 72, 75–76, 79,
  111
Vitamin B_{12}, 76
Vitamin C (ascorbic acid), 72, 77
Vitamin D, 72, 74–75
Vitamin deficiencies, 72–73, 74, 75,
  76, 77, 105–6
Vitamin E, 47, 72, 74
Vitamin K, 72, 75
Vitamins, 63, 64, 71, 72–77, 80
  supplements, 73

Vitamins (*cont'd*)
    therapy, 47, 79
Vitiligo, 170, 171–72, 173

Warts, 98, 116, 119–20, 132, 199,
    200
    venereal, 130
Waxing, 94, 95
Wens, 161
Wet dressings, 23–24
White spots, in mouth, 106–7
Whiteheads (comedones), 36, 40,
    41, 176
Wilson's disease, 103

Women
    and baldness, 87, 90
    excess hair, 93–94
Wrinkling, 8

X-ray therapy, 41–42, 94, 151, 153
X rays, 143, 165
Xerosis (winter itch), 15

Yeast fungus, 100–1
Yeast infections, 121–22

Zinc, 47, 77–78
Zinc oxide (ointment), 147